Markus Rechsteiner

Function of LMP2B in EBV-positive Burkitt's Lymphoma

Markus Rechsteiner

Function of LMP2B in EBV-positive Burkitt's Lymphoma

Virus and cancer

Südwestdeutscher Verlag für Hochschulschriften

Impressum/Imprint (nur für Deutschland/ only for Germany)
Bibliografische Information der Deutschen Nationalbibliothek: Die Deutsche Nationalbibliothek verzeichnet diese Publikation in der Deutschen Nationalbibliografie; detaillierte bibliografische Daten sind im Internet über http://dnb.d-nb.de abrufbar.
Alle in diesem Buch genannten Marken und Produktnamen unterliegen warenzeichen-, marken- oder patentrechtlichem Schutz bzw. sind Warenzeichen oder eingetragene Warenzeichen der jeweiligen Inhaber. Die Wiedergabe von Marken, Produktnamen, Gebrauchsnamen, Handelsnamen, Warenbezeichnungen u.s.w. in diesem Werk berechtigt auch ohne besondere Kennzeichnung nicht zu der Annahme, dass solche Namen im Sinne der Warenzeichen- und Markenschutzgesetzgebung als frei zu betrachten wären und daher von jedermann benutzt werden dürften.

Verlag: Südwestdeutscher Verlag für Hochschulschriften Aktiengesellschaft & Co. KG
Dudweiler Landstr. 99, 66123 Saarbrücken, Deutschland
Telefon +49 681 37 20 271-1, Telefax +49 681 37 20 271-0, Email: info@svh-verlag.de
Zugl.: Zurich, UniZH, Diss., 2008

Herstellung in Deutschland:
Schaltungsdienst Lange o.H.G., Berlin
Books on Demand GmbH, Norderstedt
Reha GmbH, Saarbrücken
Amazon Distribution GmbH, Leipzig
ISBN: 978-3-8381-0660-1

Imprint (only for USA, GB)
Bibliographic information published by the Deutsche Nationalbibliothek: The Deutsche Nationalbibliothek lists this publication in the Deutsche Nationalbibliografie; detailed bibliographic data are available in the Internet at http://dnb.d-nb.de.
Any brand names and product names mentioned in this book are subject to trademark, brand or patent protection and are trademarks or registered trademarks of their respective holders. The use of brand names, product names, common names, trade names, product descriptions etc. even without a particular marking in this works is in no way to be construed to mean that such names may be regarded as unrestricted in respect of trademark and brand protection legislation and could thus be used by anyone.

Publisher:
Südwestdeutscher Verlag für Hochschulschriften Aktiengesellschaft & Co. KG
Dudweiler Landstr. 99, 66123 Saarbrücken, Germany
Phone +49 681 37 20 271-1, Fax +49 681 37 20 271-0, Email: info@svh-verlag.de

Copyright © 2009 by the author and Südwestdeutscher Verlag für Hochschulschriften Aktiengesellschaft & Co. KG and licensors
All rights reserved. Saarbrücken 2009

Printed in the U.S.A.
Printed in the U.K. by (see last page)
ISBN: 978-3-8381-0660-1

Table of contents

1. Summary 3
2. Zusammenfassung 4
3. Introduction 6
   3.1 Tumor viruses 6
4. Epstein-Barr Virus infection and lymphomagenesis 9
   4.1 Epstein-Barr Virus 9
   4.2 Latency programs of EBV at and after primary infection 9
   4.3 Latency programs of EBV in lymphomagenesis 11
   4.4 EBV and Burkitt's lymphoma 12
   4.5 EBV and Hodgkin's lymphoma 13
   4.6 Inducers of lytic EBV infection in vitro 14
   4.7 Viral and cellular sensors for latent EBV disruption 16
5. Subject of investigation 45
6. Results 46
   6.1 Zebularine reactivates silenced E-cadherin but unlike 5-Azacytidine does not induce switching from latent to lytic Epstein-Barr virus infection in Burkitt lymphoma Akata cells 47
   6.2 Silencing of latent membrane protein 2B (LMP2B) reduces susceptibility to activation of lytic Epstein-Barr virus in Burkitt's lymphoma Akata cells 54
   6.3 Latent membrane protein 2B regulates susceptibility to activation of lytic Epstein-Barr virus infection 61
7. Discussion 71
   7.1 Induction of lytic EBV infection as treatment in clinics 71
   7.2 Induction of lytic EBV infection by LMP2B as treatment in clinics 71
8. Conclusions and outlook 73
9. Literature 74

1. Summary

Epstein-Barr virus (EBV) is a human γ-herpesvirus that, following primary infection, persists latently in the host's memory B-cell pool for life and may periodically reactivate to lytic infection. EBV is linked to malignancies including Burkitt's lymphoma (BL), Hodgkin's lymphoma (HL), and post-transplant lymphoproliferative diseases where it expresses different patterns of latency genes. Among these genes, latent membrane protein (LMP)2A and LMP2B seem to be involved in the regulation of EBV latency. LMP2A blocks the signalling from the B-cell receptor (BCR) after its engagement, which results otherwise in switching from latent to lytic EBV infection and induction of apoptosis. Therefore, LMP2A contributes to ensuring the persistence of EBV in the latently infected B-cell. By contrast, the function of LMP2B, a splice variant of LMP2A, and its interaction with LMP2A is still not resolved. Thus, the investigation of the function of LMP2B and its contribution to latent and lytic EBV infection was the main goal of my PhD thesis.

To study switching of latent to lytic EBV the EBV-harboring BL cell line Akata was employed. BL Akata cells can easily be induced to switch latent to lytic EBV upon engagement of their BCR through cross-linking using anti-human immunoglobulin antibodies. BL Akata cells with silenced *LMP2A*, silenced *LMP2B*, overexpressed LMP2A, or overexpressed LMP2B were generated.

The establishment of these cell lines revealed for the first time that silencing of *LMP2B* in EBV-harboring BL cells resulted in reduced expression of the initiator of lytic EBV, i.e., immediate-early lytic *BZLF1* EBV gene mRNA and late lytic gp350/220 protein upon BCR cross-linking. Similarly, reduction of lytic EBV activation was observed in BL Akata cells overexpressing LMP2A. By contrast, silencing of *LMP2A* and LMP2B overexpression in BL Akata cells resulted in higher lytic EBV mRNA and protein expression upon BCR cross-linking. We could further demonstrate that LMP2A and LMP2B physically interact and that LMP2B resides predominantly in intracellular compartments, whereas LMP2A was detected on the plasma membrane as well as in intracellular compartments.

In conclusion, these observations indicate a role for LMP2B distinct from LMP2A in regulation of lytic EBV activation in the host cell and support the hypothesis that LMP2B exhibits a negative regulatory effect on the ability of LMP2A to maintain latent EBV by preventing the switch to lytic EBV.

2. Zusammenfassung

Das Epstein-Barr Virus (EBV) ist ein humanes γ-Herpesvirus, welches nach der Primärinfektion eine lebenslange, latente Infektion in memory B Zellen etabliert und periodisch in seine lytische Form wechseln kann. EBV wird mit verschiedenen Malignomen assoziiert, unter anderem mit dem Burkitt's Lymphom (BL), dem Hodgkin's Lymphom (HL) und der lymphoproliferativen Krankheiten nach Organtransplantation, in denen das Virus unterschiedliche Expressionsmuster der Latenzgene aufweist. Unter diesen Genen befindet sich das Latente Membran Protein (LMP)2A und LMP2B, welche die lytische und latente Form von EBV zu regulieren scheinen. LMP2A blockiert die Signalkaskade welche vom B Zell Rezeptor nach dessen Aktivierung durch ein fremdes Antigen ausgelöst wird. Die Signalkaskade würde im Normalfall zur Induktion der lytischen Form von EBV führen und letztendlich in Apoptose enden. Deshalb stellt LMP2A die Aufrechterhaltung des latenten Zustandes von EBV sicher. Andererseits ist über die Funktion von LMP2B, einer Splicevariante von LMP2A, wenig bekannt. Das Hauptziel meines PhD Projektes war nun, die Funktion von LMP2B zu definieren und seinen Beitrag zur latenten und lytischen EBV Infektion zu untersuchen.

Um die Aktivierung von latentem zu lytischem EBV zu studieren, wurde die EBV-positive BL Zelllinie Akata verwendet. BL Akata Zellen können leicht stimuliert werden, indem der B Zell Rezeptor mit spezifischen menschlichen Immunglobulinen aktiviert wird, was zur Induktion von lytischem EBV führt. Deshalb wurden BL Akata Zellen mit gesilenztem *LMP2A*, gesilenztem *LMP2B*, überexprimiertem LMP2A und überexprimiertem LMP2B etabliert.

Diese Zelllinien ermöglichen zum ersten Mal zu demonstrieren, dass durch gesilenztes *LMP2B* die lytische Aktivierung von EBV vermindert werden konnte. Als read-out bestimmten wir die mRNA Expression des initialen lytischen EBV Genes *BZLF1* und die Proteinmenge des viralen Hüllenproteins gp350/220 nach B Zell Rezeptor Stimulation. Vergleichsweise führte die Überexpression von LMP2A zu verminderter lytischen EBV Aktivierung in BL Akata Zellen. Andersiets resultierte das Silenzing von *LMP2A* und die Überexpression von LMP2B in BL Akata Zellen nach Stimulation in höheren lytischen EBV mRNA- und Proteinlevels. Des Weiteren wurde gezeigt, dass LMP2A und LMP2B physikalisch interagieren und dass LMP2B hauptsächlich in intrazellulären Kompartimenten vorkommt, während LMP2A auf der Plasmamembran sowie in intrazellulären Kompartimenten detektiert wurde.

Diese Beobachtungen lassen auf eine unterschiedliche Rolle von LMP2B in der Regulation von lytischem und latentem EBV im Vergleich zu LMP2A schliessen und unterstützt die Hypothese, dass LMP2B einen negativ regulatorischen Effekt auf LMP2A und dessen Funktion in der Aufrechterhaltung des latenten Zustandes von EBV aufweist.

3. Introduction

3.1 Tumor viruses

Virus infection and tumor formation have been associated for the first time in 1910 by Peyton Rous. He could demonstrate that filtered cell supernatant derived from a chicken sarcoma induced new sarcoma formation in a healthy chicken. The sarcoma inducing agent was then termed Rous sarcoma virus (RSV). The identification of other viruses which induce tumor formation took almost a half of a century, i.e., the Shope virus causing papillomas in rabbits which was later found to be related to the human papilloma virus (HPV). The latter is known to cause cervical cancer, and a vaccine against HPV has most recently been licensed [1].

Intensive studies in the recent decades revealed that almost 15% of human cancers are associated to various types of viral infections, including retro-viruses, non-retroviral RNA viruses and DNA viruses [2] (Table 1). However, in many cases it is hard to pinpoint the cancer to a specific virus infection because the causal evidence can only be obtained after, e.g., immunization against a specific virus resulting in a significant reduced tumor incidence. Best reported are the vaccinations against Hepatitis B virus (HBV) for prevention of hepatocellular carcinoma or as mentioned above against HPV [1,3].

A hallmark of cancer is the continuous proliferation of cells, lacking any restrictive control of growth [4]. The outgrowth of such a cell sub-population is caused by many factors, including genetical and environmental factors, to which the virus tumors belong. Among the genetical diseases linked to cancer are hereditary mal-functions of cellular genes resulting in, e.g., loss of tumor suppressors as described in retinoblastoma or breast cancer [5,6]. However, there are more cancers associated with aberrations in somatic cells acquired during time depending on environmental factors. Among these environmental factors, infections with viruses are the second highest risk factor for cancer development after tobacco consumption [7].

The mechanisms how viruses can contribute to tumor formation are multi-faceted. Many viruses establish persistent infections and cancer may occur as an accidental side effect of the long-term interaction of the virus and the host cell [7]. Therefore, other risk factors must be taken into account, proposed as a triad function composed by viral infection, a co-carcinogen and a defective immune response leading finally to tumor formation. Furthermore, the impact of viral infections may be either indirect, by the continuous interaction of the virus and the host implicating chronic inflammation (HBV, Hepatitis C virus (HCV)), alteration of the immune response, and accumulation of mutations in infected cells or direct, manifested by the expression of viral oncogenes (*v-onc*) driving cell proliferation and malignant transformation.

Well studied viral oncogenes directly affecting cell proliferation and transformation are for example the Tax protein from the human T-cell leukemia virus 1 (HTLV-1) or the latent membrane protein(LMP)1 from Epstein-Barr virus (EBV) [8, 9].

Table 1: Characteristics of Human Oncogenic Viruses and their associated pathologies. Adapted from Boccardo and Villa.

Virus	Family/Genus	Genome	Target cell	Associated diseases	Associated cancers
Epstein-Barr Virus (EBV)	Herpesviridae/Lymphocryptovirus	dsDNA	B-lymphocytes, Oropharyngeal epithelial cells	Table 3	Table 3
Kaposi's sarcoma Herpesvirus (KSHV)	Herpesviridae/ Rhadinovirus	dsDNA	Endothelial cells, Lymphocytes	Skin lesions, Heary leukoplakia	Kaposi sarcoma
Human T-cell leukemia virus (HTLV-I)	Retroviridae/Deltaretrovirus	ssRNA	T-lymphocytes	Uveitis, Infective dermatitis	ATL
Human Immunodeficiency Virus (HIV)	Retroviridae/Lentivirus	ssRNA	CD4+ T-cells	AIDS	ARL, HD, MM
Hepatitis B Virus (HBV)	Hepadnaviridae/Orthohepadnavirus	dsDNA	Hepatocytes	Hepatitis, cirrhosis	Hepatocellular carcinoma
Hepatitis C Virus (HCV)	Flaviviridae/Hepacivirus	ssRNA	Hepatocytes	Hepatitis, cirrhosis	Hepatocellular carcinoma
Human Papillomavirus (HPV)	Papillomaviridae/k-papillomavirus	dsDNA	Mucosal and Cutaneous squamous epithelial cells	Condyloma acuminate, Common warts	Ano-genital carcinomas, cutaneous carcinoma

ATL: adult T-cell leukemia; AIDS: Acquired Immunodeficiency syndrome; ARL: AIDS related lymphomas (includes Burkitt's lymphoma, diffuse large B-cell lymphoma, Post-transplant lymphoproliferative disorder like B-cell lymphomas); HD: Hodgkin's lymphoma; MM: Multiple myeloma.

Astonishingly, EBV is present in more than 90 % of healthy individuals of the world's population [10, 11], creating an enigma about the pathology of EBV infection. EBV has been linked to non-Hodgkin's and Hodgkin's lymphomas [12] but the incidence is far below the expected malignant impact of a powerful oncogenic virus. Thus, the term of EBV as an oncogenic virus has been challenged and revised. EBV is actually one of the most successful viruses because (i) it does not kill its host cell but establishes a latent infection and (ii) the infected cells expressing oncogenic genes as LMP1 are erased by the immune system in that way preventing the outgrowth of tumors and harm to the host. This was supported by the findings that after EBV infects a B cell, initial expression of LMP1 is shut down and latency is established [13]. Furthermore, occasional switch to another viral latency state of EBV includes the expression of LMP1 with subsequent initiation of specific cytotoxic T-cell killing in healthy individuals [14]. Additionally, tumor cells containing EBV emerge in EBV positive patients after treatment with immunosuppressive drugs or in association with HIV infection reflecting the loss of immunosurveillance and the capability of malignant transformation by viral oncogenes. Thus, taken together these facts, malignancies associated with EBV infection seem to be an unwanted side effect of the virus. Nevertheless, EBV positive tumors represent a life threatening disease and host-pathogen interaction need careful investigation for effective intervention and cure.

In the following paragraphs, EBV infection and its contribution to lymphomagenesis is described.

4. Epstein-Barr Virus infection and lymphomagenesis

4.1 Epstein-Barr Virus

The Epstein-Barr virus (EBV) is a B-lymphotropic γ-herpesvirus which was discovered by the British scientists Epstein, Achong and Barr in cells cultured from endemic Burkitt's lymphoma (eBL) tissue by electron microscopy in 1964 [15]. Endemic BL was then diagnosed in more than 95 % of observed cases EBV positive and was found to be located predominantly in sub-Saharan Africa where malaria infection represents one of the major illnesses [16]. Subsequent epidemiologic investigations revealed that EBV infects more than 90% of the human population [10, 11]. Primary infection with EBV is transmitted via saliva and acquired mostly during childhood and adolescence, and may go unrecognized or manifest as infectious mononucleosis (IM), a febrile illness characterized by tonsillopharyngitis, and generally enlarged lymph nodes, liver and spleen.

4.2 Latency programs of EBV at and after primary infection

Primary infection occurs in the oropharynx where EBV replicates in epithelial and B cells. After primary infection, EBV establishes a latent infection in the memory B-cell pool where its linear DNA is circularized in the nucleus [17].

Depending on the differentiation stage of the newly infected B cell, different EBV gene expression pattern/programs can be observed (Figure 1; Table 2). The Growth program is defined as the EBV expression pattern detected when EBV infects mature/naïve B-cells (EBNA1-6 (EBV nuclear antigen), LMP1 (latent membrane protein 1), LMP2A, LMP2B, and EBERs (EBV-encoded RNA)) and drives the B-cell towards proliferation and a germinal center (GC) reaction [10]. In these GC B-cells, the Default program is predominantly switched on, comprised by the expression of EBNA1, LMP1, LMP2A, LMP2B, and EBERs which forces proliferation and differentiation to a memory B-cell. Upon completing differentiation, either from an initially infected mature/naïve or GC B-cell, the infected memory B-cells enter the periphery [10].

After establishment of a latent infection in the memory B-cell pool, EBV can be detected in 1 to 50 cells per 10^6 circulating B-cells [18, 19]. In these circulating memory B-cells, resting (Latency 0) and dividing (Latency I) memory B-cells can be distinguished by the EBV gene expression of EBERs only and EBERs, EBNA1, and occasionally LMP2A, respectively [10]. EBERs are small non-coding RNAs, which are abundantly expressed in the infected B-cell [20].

EBER1 is highly structured and inhibits protein kinase R (PKR) which is involved in the control of protein synthesis at the level of polypeptide chain initiation and cell death [21, 22]. EBNA1 is expressed for the replication of the EBV genome and the episomal segregation to the daughter cell at cell division. The function of LMP2A in the context of dividing memory B-cells is not yet fully understood.

Figure 1: Models for EBV infecting B cells in distinct differential stages

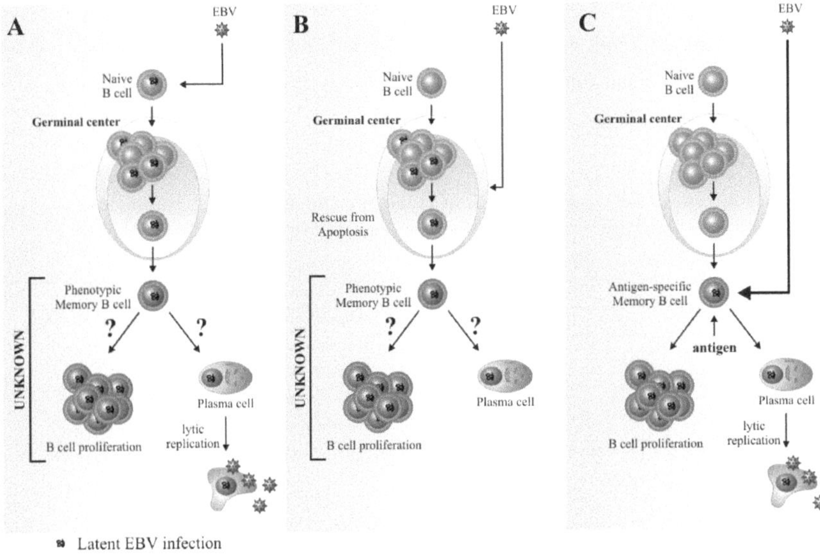

Figure 1: A: Infection of a naïve/mature B-cell with EBV. EBV initiates a germinal centre (GC) reaction and terminal differentiation into a memory B-cell. B: Direct infection of a GC B-cell by EBV and subsequent terminal differentiation into a memory B-cell. C: Direct infection of a memory B-cell by EBV. A, B, and C lead to the establishment of a latently infected memory B-cell pool. © by M. Dorner

Table 2: Patterns of EBV gene expression depending on B cell differential state

Gene expression program	EBNA1	EBNA2-6, EBNA-LP	LMP1, LMP2A, LMP2B	EBER1, EBER2	Site of infection
Growth program	+	+	+	+	Mature/naive B-cell, Epithelial cells
Default program	+		+	+	GC B-cell
Latency 0	-	-	-	+	Resting memory B-cell
Latency I	+	-	LMP2 only	+	Dividing memory B-cell

GC: germinal centre

If LMP2A is not able to rescue the activated memory B-cell due to too strong stimuli by the antigen, the lytic program of EBV is switched on. The expression of all EBV lytic genes in plasma cells leads to replication and production of new EBV particles which are released following lysis and death of the infected cell [14]. The virions are then shed in the saliva and able to infect new hosts.

4.3 Latency programs of EBV in lymphomagenesis

EBV has ever since its discovery in 1964 been associated with various lymphomas and cancers. These include lymphomas of B, T and natural killer (NK) cell origin such as the immunoblastic lymphoma of immunosuppressed, endemic Burkitt's lymphoma (BL), Hodgkin's lymphoma (HL), and nasal T/NK lymphoma, but also lymphoepitheliomas of the nasopharynx, thymus and stomach and leiomyosarcomas arising in organ transplant patients and HIV-infected individuals summarized in table 3 [12].

Table 3: Patterns of EBV gene expression in latency and associated pathologies

Latency program	EBNA1	EBNA2-6, EBNA-LP	LMP1, LMP2A, LMP2B	EBER1, EBER2	Associated cancer (EBV positivity)
Latency I	+	-	-	+	Burkitt's lymphoma (en. >95%; non-en.: 15-30%)
Latency II	+	-	+	+	Hodgkin's lymphoma (mc: 70%; ld: >95%; ns: 10-40%)
					Nasopharyngeal carcinoma (>95%)
					Peripheral T/NK lymphoma (> 90%)
Latency III	+	+	+	+	AIDS-associated lymphomas (> 90%)
					Post-transplant lymphoproliverative disorders (>90%)

EBNA, EBV nuclear antigen; LP, latent protein; LMP, latent membrane protein; EBER, EBV non-polyadenylated RNA; mc: mixed cellularity; ld: lymphocyte depleted; nc: nodular sclerosing

Not all latent EBV genes are always simultaneously expressed in the different pathological situations. Three distinct expression patterns seem to allow EBV to manipulate the host cell which lead to the formation of lymphomas or cancer while escaping immune recognition by the host [23, 24]. The Latency I program is found in BL where the only EBV genes expressed are EBNA1 and the EBERs. This EBV expression pattern resembles the one detected in dividing memory B-cells of healthy carriers as described in Table 2. The Latency II program expresses EBNA1 plus LMP1, LMP2A, LMP2B, and EBERs and is associated with HL, nasopharyngeal carcinoma (NPC), and peripheral T/NK lymphoma [12]. The Latency III program involves expression of all six EBNAs, the LMPs (1, 2A, 2B), and EBERs and is found in immunocompromized hosts including posttransplant lymphoproliferative diseases (PTLD) and AIDS-associated lymphomas [25]. As EBV latency III resembles the EBV expression pattern of the Growth program it would normally elicit T-cell response and eradication of the tumorigenic memory B-cells. Thus, in individuals with an intact immune system no EBV-positive B-cells expressing Latency III are detected.

4.4 EBV and Burkitt's lymphoma

The hallmark of all BLs is the reciprocal translocation of *c-myc* and an immunoglobulin gene, most often between chromosomes 8 and 14, which places *c-myc* under the control of Ig transcription-controlling promoter and enhancer sequences [26]. This translocation leads to a continuous high expression of *c-myc* in B-cells, driving proliferation and favours tumor formation. Cells normally undergo apoptosis when c-myc reaches a certain threshold [27]. Thus, there is a selection for other mutations, abrogating the apoptosis-inducing signals. Such mutations are found in direct p53 inactivation or in other key players involved in the p53 pathway [28, 29].

The role of EBV in pathogenesis of BL has been widely discussed. Although *c-myc* translocation is the major event leading to tumor formation, it seems that EBV favours the translocation. There have been reports of EBV increasing genomic instability [30-33]. Moreover, EBV starts its 'Growth program' after infecting a B cell, which increases proliferation rates, allowing fast replication cycles in the initial infection before shutting-down its gene expression and establishment of the latent infected B-cell pool. Additionally, EBV increases the probability of translocations on the one hand by the initiation of a GC reaction and on the other hand in the prevention of lytic EBV infection in activated memory B-cells encountering their specific antigen in the periphery, both inducing higher proliferation rates. According to the infection of B-cells in distinct differentiation states described above, there are as well reports of BL biopsies which comprise B cells phenotypically linked to GC or memory B-cells.

Concerning these facts, BL might be derived from a memory B-cell in which EBV is found in its Latency state I as described above. Thus, it represents a model to study infected, dividing memory B-cells and the pathology of EBV controlling the switch from latent to lytic EBV infection. Due to the fact that the BL cell line Akata shows adequate activation of lytic EBV infection after BCR cross-linking with anti-IgG [34, 35], this cell line is an optimal model system as close as possible to the *in vivo* situation for investigating the impact of LMP2A and LMP2B in the maintenance of latent and lytic EBV infection.

Endemic BL accounts for up to 74 % of childhood malignancies in the African equatorial belt where it is as well associated with malaria infection [26, 36]. Whereas endemic BL is in most cases comprised of EBV positive B cells, sporadic BL contains in 15-30 % of the cases EBV positive tumor cells (Table 3). BL characteristically involves the jaw or other facial bones, ovaries, kidney or the breast. Because of the rapid rate of tumor growth in BL, it is important to begin treatment as soon as possible after diagnosis. Bulky abdominal tumors or chest tumors are sometimes removed surgically before the patient begins chemotherapy or radiation therapy. Untreated BL is often followed by rapid death of the patient. Today, BL is treated with a short course of high-dose chemotherapy, usually with cyclophosphamide (Endoxan), a drug that is converted *in vivo* into two active compounds which interfere with DNA and replication, in combination of methotrexate (purine and pyrimidine synthesis inhibitor), vincristine (mitotic spindle formation inhibitor), prednisone (steroid; immunosuppressive), and doxorubicin (replication inhibitor; DNA intercalating).

The sensibility of BL to combination chemotherapies is greater the more localized the tumor is. Once the tumor expanded to the bone marrow or the central nervous system (CNS) the cure rate decreases dramatically. Although the cytotoxic drugs exhibit collateral effects by killing healthy cells, the cure rate nowadays is more than 50%.

4.5 EBV and Hodgkin's lymphoma

HL is a type of lymphoma first described by Thomas Hodgkin in 1832 defined as a malignant disorder in which there is progressive (but painless) enlargement of lymph tissue followed by enlargement of the spleen and liver. HL can be divided into four subtypes defined by their histological pattern which are summarized in table 3. HL is characterized clinically by spread of disease from one lymph node to another and by the development of systemic symptoms as fever or weight loss. The incidence of new HL arising a year lies between 2 and 4 per 100'000 inhabitants. The tumor of HL comprises only about 1-2% malignant cells which are named Reed Sternberg cells (RSC). The fast majority of the tumor mass is from cells activated due to continuous inflammation and cytokine secretion, i.e., macrophages, T-cells, and granulocytes. The RSCs are derived from B cells. Due to the fact, that only 1-2 % of tumor cells are responsible for the tumor formation, the isolation and characterization of these cells has been extremely difficult. Recently, it has been postulated that EBV associated HL contains B-cells with crippled and non-functional BCRs which then result in the malignant RSCs [37, 38]. Moreover, the RSCs in HL were defined by their surface immunoglobulin expression pattern, as GC B-cells and due to viral LMP2A, LMP2B and LMP1 expression to belong to the EBV Latency program II. For more detailed information how LMP2A and LMP2B are interconnected with HL, please refer to section 4.7.

HL was one of the first cancers to be cured by radiation and subsequently by combination chemotherapy. Currently, *ABVD* chemotherapy is the gold standard for treatment of HL. The abbreviation stands for the four drugs doxorubicin, bleomycin (induction of DNA strand brakes), vinblastine (mitotic inhibitor), and dacarbazine (alkylating DNA agent). The cure rate is about 93%, making it one of the most curable forms of cancer.

4.6 Inducers of lytic EBV infection in vitro

Activation of the lytic infection can be initiated by a variety of agents in culture, including anti-immunoglobulin, calcium ionophore, sodium-butyrate and the phorbol ester 12-O-tetradecanyl-phorbol-13-acetate (TPA) summarized in Table 4. These agents exhibit considerable variability in the degree of activation of lytic EBV infection in established EBV-infected cell lines. Anti-IgG, as described above, and anti-IgM stimulation showed a high activation of lytic EBV infection in the BL cell lines Akata and Ramos, respectively [34]. Induction of lytic EBV infection using various compounds including 5-Azacytidine and dexamethasone is increasingly being explored as a potential treatment of EBV-carrying malignancies, but the use of these compounds may be burdened or limited by toxic side effects [39-42].

Table 4: Inducers of lytic EBV infection *in vitro*

Agent	Mode of action	Reference
anti-immunoglobulin	BCR cross-linking	35, 43
calcium ionophore A23187	Calcium flux induction	44
Doxorubicin	DNA interference	44, 45
cis-platin	DNA interference	44
Methotrexate	Metabolic inhibitor	46
Gemcitabine	Cytidine analogue	45
TPA	Phorbol ester; PKC activator	43
TGF-β	Not known	43
Dexamethasone	Glucocorticoid	40
5-Azacytidine	DNMTI	11, 47, 48
sodium-butyrate	Histone deacetylase inhibitor	11, 48
Trichostatin A	Histone deacetylase inhibitor	49

TPA: 12-O- tetradecanyl-phorbol-13-acetate; DNMTI: DNA methyl transferase inhibitor

Among the DNA methyl transferase inhibitors (DNMTI), the recently discovered Zebularine is the most promising. The advantages of Zebularine lies in its long half-life and stability [50, 51]. Additionally, it is well tolerated in far higher concentrations than for example the more toxic 5-Azacytidine [52]. Moreover, it has been demonstrated that its administration switches silenced genes on by demethylation and kills specifically tumor cells [53]. Thus, the impact of Zebularine on EBV infected BL cells might represent a powerful tool as the genome of EBV in BLs is hypermethylated. Demethylation might lead to lytic EBV infection resulting in tumor cell death.

4.7 Viral and cellular sensors for latent EBV disruption

Manuscript in preparation

Markus P. Rechsteiner, Mark Rovedo, Michele Bernasconi, Richard Longnecker, Christoph Berger, and David Nadal

Abstract

The oncogenic Epstein-Barr virus (EBV) infects the majority of the human population and establishes a life-long latent infection in B cells from which the virus may reactivate periodically. To cope with these prerequisites, EBV hijacks B-cell differentiation pathways using on the one hand own viral genes interfering with B-cell signalling to establish latent infection for life-long persistence and on the other hand cellular genes as sensors for the switch of latent to lytic EBV infection. A prominent protein is the viral latent membrane protein (LMP)2A which is believed to play a crucial role in the maintenance of latent EBV by blocking activation of its host cell and by providing a surrogate B-cell receptor (BCR) signal essential for cell survival [1, 2]. These two functions of LMP2A demand a tight control of LMP2A activity and expression levels. Recent insights in LMP2B [3-5], an isoform of LMP2A, prompt us to hypothesize that LMP2B modulates the activity of LMP2A and regulates in that way activation of lytic EBV infection. Another gene terminating latent EBV infection is the cellular factor X-box binding protein (XBP)-1 which is upregulated during terminal plasma cell differentiation and increases the transcription of the master EBV lytic regulator gene *BZLF1* [6, 7]. In this review we summarize the latest findings of EBV hijacking the normal B-cell differentiation pathways.

Viral and cellular sensors for latent EBV disruption

Markus P. Rechsteiner,[1] Mark Rovedo,[2] Michele Bernasconi,[1] Richard Longnecker,[2] Christoph Berger,[1] and David Nadal[1]

[1] Experimental Infectious Diseases and Cancer Research, Division of Infectious Diseases and Hospital Epidemiology, University Children's Hospital of Zurich, CH-8032 Zurich, Switzerland, and [2]Department of Microbiology and Immunology, Feinberg School of Medicine, Northwestern University, Chicago, Illinois 60611.

The oncogenic Epstein-Barr virus (EBV) infects the majority of the human population and establishes a life-long latent infection in B cells from which the virus may reactivate periodically. To cope with these prerequisites, EBV hijacks B-cell differentiation pathways using on the one hand own viral genes interfering with B-cell signalling to establish latent infection for life-long persistence and on the other hand cellular genes as sensors for the switch of latent to lytic EBV infection. A prominent protein is the viral latent membrane protein (LMP)2A which is believed to play a crucial role in the maintenance of latent EBV by blocking activation of its host cell and by providing a surrogate B-cell receptor (BCR) signal essential for cell survival [1, 2]. These two functions of LMP2A demand a tight control of LMP2A activity and expression levels. Recent insights in LMP2B [3-5], an isoform of LMP2A, prompt us to hypothesize that LMP2B modulates the activity of LMP2A and regulates in that way activation of lytic EBV infection. Another gene terminating latent EBV infection is the cellular factor X-box binding protein (XBP)-1 which is upregulated during terminal plasma cell differentiation and increases the transcription of the master EBV lytic regulator gene *BZLF1* [6, 7]. In this review we summarize the latest findings of EBV hijacking the normal B-cell differentiation pathways.

Epstein–Barr virus (EBV) is a ubiquitous human gammaherpesvirus linked to many malignancies including Burkitt's lymphoma (BL) and Hodgkin's lymphoma (HL) [8, 9]. After primary infection, EBV enters the memory B-cell pool establishing a life-long latent infection from which lymphomas might arise [1, 10]. Once in its latent form, EBV persists as an episome in the nucleus. The EBV genome is maintained by segregation of its episome to the daughter cell after mitotic cell division. Occasionally, there is activation of lytic EBV infection which leads to the production of infectious particles and host cell death. EBV hijacks B cells at specific stages of B-cell differentiation and uses on the one hand own viral genes for manipulation of signalling pathways in the B cell and on the other hand cellular genes as sensors for the switch of latent to lytic EBV infection. Whether these rare events of activation are triggered by the virus, host cell factors, or both acting synergistically remains to be resolved.

In this review, we will focus on the viral gene *LMP2* and the cellular gene *XBP-1* and their impact on B-cell differentiation pathways and latent and lytic EBV infection. Moreover, we will especially pay regard to the expression of LMP2B and LMP2A in different cellular compartments, propose a model of interaction and regulation of each other, and outline their possible functions in B-cell differentiation.

1. EBV: hijacker of B-cell differentiation pathways

EBV hijacks B cells at specific stages of B-cell differentiation and uses on the one hand own viral genes for manipulation of signalling pathways in the B cell and on the other hand viral and cellular genes as sensors for the switch of latent to lytic EBV infection.

B-cell development can be divided into three main stages depending on localization [11]: (i) primary lymphoid tissue (bone marrow), (ii) germinal centre, and (iii) blood and secondary lymphoid tissue. The B cells present in the bone marrow can be further subdivided into pro-, and pre- B-cells. Pro- B-cells undergo heavy and pre- B-cells light chain B-cell receptor (BCR) rearrangements. After functional rearrangement and BCR expression on the surface, the B cell is termed as mature or naïve and is released into the blood stream. Once encountering an antigen either in the blood or presented in lymph nodes by follicular dendritic cells (fDCs) where the mature/naïve B-cells pass by from time to time, there occurs together with T helper cells the formation of a follicle with germinal centres (GC). In the the GC reaction, B-cells with high affinity for a specific antigen are produced by somatic hypermutation. The activated and hypermutated B-cells can then either differentiate into antibody secernating plasma cells or enter the memory B-cell pool.

A prominent viral gene hijacking B-cell differentiation pathways encodes for the latent membrane protein (LMP) 2A. LMP2A exploits the BCR signalling pathway generating a tonic signal which is needed for B-cell survival with crippled BCRs or for the initiation of the germinal centre (GC) reaction. Another prerequisite of LMP2A represents the regulation of latent and lytic EBV infection by blocking BCR signalling induced by binding of an antigen. These apparently opposite functions of LMP2A, on the one hand producing tonic BCR survival signals and on the other hand blocking BCR signal [1,2], leads to the question how this dual function is achieved. Recent findings suggest specific functions of LMP2A depending on its protein levels present in the host cell. Furthermore, there is evidence that LMP2A levels are influenced and regulated by its isoform LMP2B which may influence the carefully maintained balance of host cell survival and lytic EBV infection described more in detail in section 2-5 [3-5].

Another pathway in B-cell differentiation hijacked by EBV has recently been described. The cellular factor X-box binding protein (XBP)-1 was suggested as initiator of ultimately terminating latent EBV infection [6,7]. XBP-1 is active in plasma cells and increases the transcription of the master EBV lytic regulator gene *BZLF1*, which leads to the production of new infectious virions. This interesting finding links activation of lytic EBV directly to terminal B-cell differentiation into a plasma cell which is outlined in section 6.

2. Epstein-Barr virus LMP2B: a rheostat for LMP2A signal strength

The *LMP2* gene is transcribed into two mRNAs across the circularized EBV genome (i.e., across the terminal repeats) from two spatially distinct promoter elements. Both transcripts are multiply spliced and exons 2–9 are shared by both mRNAs. Exon 1 of *LMP2A* encodes a hydrophilic, N-terminal cytoplasmic domain of 119 amino acids, whereas exon 1 of *LMP2B* is non-coding, with translation beginning in the common exon 2 before the first transmembrane sequence [12-14]. The remaining exons encode 12 transmembrane domains and a 27 aa, hydrophilic C terminus [12, 14]. The molecular characteristics of LMP2A were recently reviewed by Brinkmann and Schulz [15]. Since LMP2B is lacking the N-terminal domain, it has been postulated that interaction between LMP2A and LMP2B occurs via their C-termini [16]. The expression of both isoforms together, LMP2A and LMP2B, was detected in HL and nasopharyngeal carcinoma (NPC) biopsies as well as in EBV-positive post-transplant-lymphoproliferative diseases (PTLDs) and in *in vitro* transformed B-cells (lymphoblastoid cell lines (LCLs)) [17-21]. The expression of LMP2A alone was detected only in peripheral blood memory B-cells [22] and in BL cells stimulated either by B-cell receptor (BCR) cross-linking or with chemical agents or biologicals including TPA, TGF-β, or 5-Azacytidine [23-29].

The regulation of LMP2A levels has been addressed in various publications and its need for differential expression levels seems to be evident for B-cells [30-35]. Portis and co-workers suggested a regulation of LMP2A by ubiquitination [34]. They proposed a model where ubiquitin protein ligase present in the cell is dependent on the levels of Notch. Notch is a transmembranal protein, which is cleaved upon binding to an extracellular ligand, releasing its intracellular part (NotchIC) for entering the nucleus [36-38]. Once in the nucleus Notch activates RBP-Jk/CBF-1 which is involved in the regulation of many genes, among them genes important for lymphocyte development. As Notch and LMP2A are ubiquitinated by the same protein ligases, Portis and co-workers proposed that Notch sequesters the ligases in similar manner as LMP2A sequesters Scr kinases from the BCR complex [15] and thereby prevents ubiquitination dependent degradation of LMP2A. In other words, high protein levels of LMP2A result in ubiquitin-mediated degradation and the increase of Notch, and vice versa. This conclusion is supported by the fact that in HL, where LMP2A is expressed constitutively and sequesters ubiquitin ligases continuously, high Notch levels have been detected [39]. Recently, it was shown that LMP2A influences Notch protein levels which in turn enhance transcription of LMP2A in B-cells and epithelial cells [40]. Thus, LMP2A seems to control its expression levels via an auto-regulatory loop. However, through which pathway Notch is upregulated remains elusive. Taken together upregulation of LMP2A leads to a positive feedback loop on transcriptional and protein level.

Observations that LMP2B modulates the activity of LMP2A [5] and influences the induction of lytic EBV [3, 4] suggest that LMP2B is an important key player in regulating LMP2A's degradation or LMP2A's auto-regulatory loop. Thus, these findings prompted us to hypothesize that EBV modulates the protein levels of LMP2B to control the activity and/or protein levels of LMP2A and the strength of the BCR signal.

If the question is asked, whether LMP2B is a rheostat of LMP2A signal strength, an important prerequisite is, in which cellular compartment LMP2B interacts with and regulates the activity of LMP2A. There have been several reports on the localization of untagged and tagged LMP2B and LMP2A [3-5, 41-47] (Table 1). Both isoforms localize in different cellular compartments depending on the host cell. In B-cells with or without EBV, LMP2B shifted to intracellular compartments as perinuclear regions and the trans Golgi network (TGN) whereas LMP2A was found on the plasma membrane as well as in intracellular regions [3-5, 42-46] (Table 1). In epithelial cells, including those in NPC biopsies, LMP2B and LMP2A were detected in the plasma membrane and intracellular regions [41, 43, 45-48] (Table 1). It has been shown that LMPB and LMP2A can interact physically and that the C-terminus shared by both isoforms contributes mainly for the clustering [4, 16]. The protein domains which seem to be important for LMP2B localization and the ability to cluster with itself or heterodimerize with LMP2A were mapped to the transmembranal loops of LMP2B [47].

LMP2B might regulate the activity of LMP2A in B-cells in different ways: as described in Figure 1, depending on the amount of newly translated LMP2A and LMP2B, the two isoforms may either homodimerize or heterodimerize in the TGN. The prevalence for dimerization lies in the expression levels of both proteins and is an important prerequisite for the regulation of BCR signalling.

When high amounts of LMP2A are translated, they homodimerize already in the TGN. However, as Syk, Lyn, and Nedd4 ubiquitin ligases are not or only in small amounts present in the TGN, LMP2A cannot sequester Scr kinases and ubiquitin ligases which would lead to ubiquitination and degradation of the participating proteins in proteasomes. Thus, vesicles containing LMP2A are able to traffic from the TGN to the plasma membrane where they fuse. After localizing to the plasma membrane, homodimerized LMP2A gets activated by phosphorylation. Upon activation, LMP2A assembles a signalosome in lipid rafts comprised of Scr kinases and ubiquitin ligases [49]. This scenario is supported by the finding that constitutively expressed LMP2A is predominantly detected in lipid rafts on plasma membranes [16, 50-52]. However, recruitment of ubiquitin ligases leads to monoubiquitination of the members of the signalosome which in turn leads to internalization into endosomes [43, 53, 54]. Depending on the state of ubiquitination, the fate of a protein is either to be reconstituted by a turn-over to the plasma membrane when monoubiquitinated or to be degraded in proteasomes when polyubiquitinated [55].

As LMP2B is detected in intracellular compartments (Table 1) it might be possible that endocytosed signalosomes and vesicles containing LMP2B fuse. This would allow the disruption of the homodimerized LMP2A by LMP2B and the rescue of LMP2A and Scr kinases by deubiquinating enzymes (DUBs) [56] resulting in an intact turn-over process and proper BCR signal once triggered by a specific antigen. On the other hand, if there occurs no fusion with a LMP2B containing vesicle, the members of the endocytosed signalosome get degraded in proteasomes and BCR signalling cannot be realized.

As depicted in figure 1, shifting from high LMP2A levels to medium amounts of LMP2A and LMP2B in the B-cell, the isoforms can heterodimerize in the TGN and traffic in vesicles to the plasma membrane. Thus, Scr kinases and ubiquitin ligases do not assemble with LMP2A to a signalosome resulting in enough Syk and Lyn present in the system for proper BCR signalling once triggered by an antigen. This scenario is supported by the fact, that transient LMP2B expression in EBV negative BL BJAB cells overexpressing LMP2A restores Lyn levels and Ca^{2+} mobilization upon cross-linking which verified proper BCR signalling. Similarly, LMP2B abrogated the effect of LMP2A blocking BCR signalling in EBV-positive Akata cells overexpressing LMP2A [57].

Once the heterodimer consisting of LMP2A and LMP2B has fused with the plasma membrane, there can occur a reorganisation of dimers as the plasma membrane and its proteins is a dynamic layer where aggregation as well as separation of proteins happen continuously. Thus, disassembly and reassembly of heterodimers to homodimers might occur, leading either to LMP2A homodimers which in turn are endocytosed as described above, or to LMP2B homodimers. Whether LMP2B homodimerization in the plasma membrane has a physiological function in the B cell is highly hypothetical. Due to the fact that LMP2B dimers do not recruit Scr kinases and ubiquitin ligases, they do not get ubiquitinated and endocytosed. This would lead to an accumulation of LMP2B in the plasma membrane. However, as LMP2A levels may be upregulated, the excess of LMP2B could act as a buffer till a threshold concentration of LMP2A in the plasma membrane is reached and BCR signalling is blocked again.

To complete the scenario described in Figure 1, the fate of high levels of LMP2B favouring homodimers in the TGN has to be addressed. In a recent publication, Tomaszewski-Flick and co-workers identified protein domains in LMP2B which, when deleted, allowed LMP2B to traffic to the plasma membrane [47]. This implicates a retention domain in LMP2B. However, as LMP2A contains the same domains as LMP2B but is detected on the plasma membrane, the retention signal seems to be inactive or overridden, probably due to another dominant signal in the additional N-terminus. Whether LMP2B homodimers traffic from the TGN to the plasma membrane or LMP2B dimers can only be formed by reassembly as described above remains elusive and needs further investigations.

Table 1: Sub-cellular localization of LMP2

Cell line	Expression	Sub-cellular localization	Reference
BL Akata	LMP2B	Predominantly intracellular regions	4
BL Akata	LMP2A	Plasma membrane and intracellular regions	3, 4
BL BJAB	LMP2A and LMP2B	Plasma membrane and intracellular regions	5
BL BJAB	LMP2A and ΔLMP2A	Plasma membrane	44
BL BJAB	LMP2A and LMP2B	Perinuclear intracellular regions / TGN	46
LCL	LMP2A	Perinuclear intracellular regions / TGN	46
LCL	LMP2A	Plasma membrane	45
LCL	LMP2A and ΔLMP2A	Plasma membrane and intracellular regions	42
LCL	LMP2A	Plasma membrane and intracellular regions	43
HEK 293T	LMP2A and LMP2B	Perinuclear intracellular regions / TGN	46
HEK 293T	LMP2B	Intracellular regions	47
HEK 293T	Various ΔLMP2B	Plasma membrane	47
BALB 3T3	LMP2A	Plasma membrane and intracellular regions	45
A321, SCC12F, HaCat	LMP2A and LMP2B	Perinuclear vesicles	41
NPC biopsies	LMP2A	Plasma membrane and intracellular regions	48

LMP2A: Latent membrane protein 2A; LMP2B: Latent membrane protein 2B; BL: Burkitt's lymphoma; LCL: lymphoblastoid cell line; Δ: deletion constructs; NPC: Nasopharyngeal carcinoma; TGN: trans-Golgi network

The proposed model of LMP2A and LMP2B in the different cellular compartments points out the importance of a very carefully regulated balance of the two isoforms. Increase of LMP2A or LMP2B protein levels shifts the balance either to a blocked or to an intact BCR signal upon antigen encounter, respectively. Due to the fact that only LMP2A can directly interfere with BCR signalling prompted us to propose LMP2B functioning as a rheostat for LMP2A signal strength. However, as the function of LMP2B *in vivo* is not yet revealed, we tried to integrate the proposed interaction between LMP2A and LMP2B depending on the stage of B-cell differentiation and nature of B-cell lymphoproliferative diseases into a model described in the following paragraphs and Figure 2.

3. LMP2B and LMP2A: effects on B-cell differentiation at the germinal centre

There is a consensus in the scientific community that EBV targets epithelial cells and B cells in the oropharynx in primary infection [58]. As it has been shown that EBV particles shed by epithelial cells infect B-cells to a higher rate and vice versa [59, 60], the first step of infection is production of a huge amount of virions. However, during productive replication, EBV expresses the whole repertoire of latent and lytic genes which leads to activation of the immune system [61]. Whereas there is clearance of EBV positive epithelial cells by cytotoxic T-cells [61], there occurs a shut down of the expression of EBV genes in B-cells, enabling the establishment of a latently infected memory B-cell pool [62].

Which B-cell subpopulations are infected by EBV has been an open field for discussion for many years. It has been long thought that only mature/naïve B-cells can be infected directly by EBV, first enhancing their proliferation and then differentiation leading through a 'pseudo' germinal centre (GC) reaction and getting access to the memory B-cell pool [21, 63]. Recently, a model has been proposed in which the direct infection of GC B-cell is considered [64]. This site of infection was then as well linked to the pathogenesis of HL, where the RSCs show surface expression markers characteristic for GC B-cells [65]. RSCs analysed so far showed crippled BCR rearrangement and the specific latency program II of EBV where LMP2A is expressed and is thought to deliver the tonic survival signal otherwise produced by the functional BCR [66]. However, we can only speculate about why the RSBs retain their GC B-cell characteristic and do not switch to memory B-cell phenotype. It might be that, although LMP1 is expressed and mimics the differentiation signal from CD40, the strength of the LMP2A signal is too low for an activated BCR in positive selection and therefore the GC B-cell is stock in its differentiation stage.

The possible role of LMP2B in GC B-cells directly infected by EBV might be that when positive selection with somatic hypermutation is induced by the binding of a foreign antigen to the BCR, the signal of LMP2A has to be regulated (Figure 2A). In the case of somatic hypermutation generating high affinity B-cells the presence of LMP2A would lead to a decrease of the signal due to less Scr kinases present in the lipid rafts, and possibly to induction of apoptosis. Thus, LMP2B might be expressed to downregulate the activity of LMP2A to allow the GC B-cell to enter the memory B-cell pool. On the other hand, when low affinity BCR rearrangements would lead to depletion of a B cell, the additional signal of LMP2A would enhance BCR signalling resulting in a high affinity signal and positive selection, as previously proposed [63, 67-69]. Therefore, memory B-cells circulating in the periphery with low affinity to a foreign antigen are generated, in that way weakening the adaptive immune response. However, whether a B-cell with low or high affinity for a foreign antigen is generated, there exists the possibility that during the GC reaction other translocations or mutations occur. Such genetic unfavourable hits include the translocation of *c-myc* and the malfunction of p53, both together leading to the phenotype of BL more closely described in section 5.

A model where EBV directly infects memory B-cells has been proposed (Dorner et al. accepted for publication in JV) [70, 71]. Tonsillar mature and memory B-cells are infected *ex vivo* at similar frequencies. In contrast, memory B-cells from blood, which represent B-cells from various lymphoid tissues, are infected at lower frequencies than their mature counterparts. According to this model EBV exploits the B-cell differentiation status and tissue of origin to establish persistent infection. Whether EBV infects B cells in various differentiation status or mature naïve B-cells only as emphasized by Souza and co-workers [63], our model proposed in Figure 2 allows the integration of the regulatory function of LMP2B on LMP2A signal strength independently of the step of infection.

4. LMP2B and LMP2A: effects on B-cell differentiation in the bone marrow

One major function of LMP2A is to deliver survival signals when EBV infects B-cells with non-functional heavy or light chain rearrangement [1, 67]. This survival signal is generated by mimicking a tonic signal otherwise produced by the BCR using its cytosolic N-terminal domain recruiting the Scr kinases Syk and Lyn [2]. The ability of EBV to enhance survival of death-doomed B cells and to access in that way the memory B-cell pool by the expression of LMP2A was underlined in *in vivo* models in RAG deficient [31] or ΔITAM-LMP2A transgenic mice [35]. These experiments were done in mice with LMP2A integrated into the germline and show the rescue capability of LMP2A signalling in B-cells with non-functional BCRs. To translate this scenario into a human background, one has to assume that EBV infects pro- and pre- B-cells in the bone marrow. Indeed, there has been a publication detecting several EBV-positive lymphoid cells on EBER-1 in situ hybridization (ISH) [72]. However, as pro- and pre- B-cells do not express CD21, the cellular surface receptor interacting with EBV's gp350 envelope protein, the attachment and entry of EBV into these cells remains elusive. In the following paragraphs we suggest a possible impact of LMP2A and LMP2B assumed that EBV infects the B-cells present in the human bone marrow.

As in the bone marrow heavy and light BCR chains are rearranged, there is always a high amount of B-cells produced with non-functional BCRs. A possible outcome of B-cells with crippled BCR is the formation of HL where only a small subset of the tumour mass, the Reed-Sternberg cells (RSCs), is accounted for the pathological situation [65, 73]. It could be shown that the RSCs indeed have crippled BCRs and that LMP2A is expressed among other latent EBV genes defined as Latency II [66, 74-78]. The RSCs resemble GC B-cells which suggests EBV infection of either mature B-cells, driving them into proliferation and differentiation to the GC reaction, or the direct infection of GC B-cells, rescuing malfunctional switch of heavy chain as well as low affinity or dysfunctional hypermutations of the variable regions [10]. Additionally, this model allows the possibility of EBV infection of pro- and pre- B-cells with crippled BCRs which would be depleted by induction of apoptosis in the bone marrow.

As in the bone marrow not only B cells with crippled BCRs are depleted but also B-cells with BCRs binding to a self-antigen, this rises the question about what happens to pro- and pre B-cells infected with EBV and a BCR-recognising self-antigen. In this scenario LMP2A would have to block the strong signal induced by the BCR/self-antigen complex. This leads to the hypothesis that LMP2A sequesters the Scr kinases Syk and Lyn and the Nedd4 ubiquitin protein ligases AIP4/Itchy, WWP2, Nedd4, and Nedd4-2/KIAA0439 [53, 54]. This constellation of the signalosome leads to ubiquitination and degradation of Lyn as was previously reported

[32, 34, 53, 79]. The situation in blocking the BCR signal due to low Lyn levels would be the same as observed in LCLs with high levels of endogenous LMP2A [79], BJAB BL cells overexpressing LMP2A [5], and BL Akata cells overexpressing LMP2A (unpublished results). The survival of B-cells recognizing self-antigen results in an increased memory B-cell pool of autoreactive B-cells of the subtype B1 [33, 80]. Generation of elevated numbers of autoreactive B-cells by EBV was discussed in the literature and is proposed to be linked with autoimmune diseases such as multiple sclerosis, rheumatoid arthritis, and systemic lupus erythematosus [69, 81-85].

With our hypothesis described in section 2 and Figure 1, it is as well possible to explain the survival of B-cells, from pro-B-cell state till mature B-cell, which have undergone functional BCR rearrangement, do not recognize self-antigen, and are infected with EBV. In these B-cells, defined as subgroup B2 [33, 80], the functional BCR provides the tonic survival signal already and LMP2A is not needed for any intervention or help. Thus, the ability of LMP2A to either provide at low levels a tonic signal or at high levels to block BCR signalling is abolished by the presence of LMP2B which disrupts homodimerization of LMP2A and its activity.

5. LMP2B and LMP2A: effects on maintenance of latent EBV infection

In order to exploit the memory B-cell pool in healthy individuals as the reservoir for latent EBV infection, there must be a tight control of viral gene expression and lytic EBV activation to avoid recognition by the immune system. The set of viral genes expressed in resting memory B-cells is restricted to the non-coding EBERs which cannot be sensed by the immune system and is defined as Latency 0 [1, 10, 86]. The stealth strategy of EBV allows the virus to survive without recognition by the innate or adaptive immune system and to establish latent infection in more than 90 % of the world population [87]. However, the handicap of the stealth strategy is that EBV replicates only when its host-cell divide. The proper replication and segregation of the EBV genomes is warranted by the expression of EBNA1 which acts in *cis* and is detected in dividing memory B-cells (Latency I) [10]. Another viral gene detected in dividing memory B-cells, although very rarely, is LMP2A [22, 88]. LMP2A blocks the signal after BCR cross-linking in *in vitro* transformed LCLs [89] and it is assumed that LMP2A exerts a similar function *in vivo* in memory B-cells that have encountered their specific antigen. This suggests a pivotal role of LMP2A in the maintenance of latent EBV infection.

This *in vivo* scenario is substantiated by an *in vitro* model using the EBV-positive BL cell line Akata [3, 4, 90]. The advantage of the BL cell line Akata is, that it retains the EBV expression pattern found in biopsies when cultured (Latency I) whereas other BL cell lines switch with time to Latency III, characteristically expressing the EBV genes EBNA1-6, LMP1, LMP2A, and LMP2B [91]. Apart from a *c-myc* translocation which is found in most BL cell lines [91], Akata cells exhibit a functional IgG rearrangement and hypermutation, therefore representing an optimal model to study EBV infected dividing memory B-cells [90]. We and others have observed the upregulation of LMP2A 48-72 h after BCR cross-linking in Akata cells which might indicate an attempted rescue of latent infection [3, 92, 93]. Thus, we investigated the impact of either silenced or overexpressed LMP2A or LMP2B on lytic EBV infection in Akata cells after BCR cross-linking [3, 4]. This Akata model system revealed that lytic EBV infection either increased after BCR cross-linking compared to control cells when LMP2B was overexpressed or LMP2A was silenced, or conversely decreased when LMP2B was silenced or LMP2A was overexpressed. These findings underscored the function of LMP2A *in vivo* as described above and elucidated a potential function of its isoform LMP2B, namely to act as a rheostat for LMP2A signal strength.

Activated memory B-cells differentiate into antibody producing plasma cells [6]. This differentiation step leads to the activation of lytic EBV infection with expression of lytic and latent viral genes, among them LMP2A [92], which triggers cytotoxic T-cell (CTL) response.

Recently published data report a decline in CTLs against immediate early viral antigenes but no decline specific for latent antigens [94]. This observation might be limited because as read-out of CTLs against latent antigenes only EBNA3C was measured. Therefore, whether LMP2A is expressed and triggers an CTL response which kills all activated EBV-positive B-cells trying to escape terminal plasma cell differentiation as desribed below remains elusive. However, according to the model described in paragraph 2 and Figure 1, the upregulation of LMP2A leads to a depletion of Scr kinases and a block of BCR signal. As the activation and differentiation of memory B-cell takes several days *in vivo* [95-98], there might be enough time for EBV to act against plasma cell fate and disruption of EBV latency with the upregulation of LMP2A according to Figure 2B and the model described in Figure 1. If this occurs, these memory B-cells rescued from plasma cell differentiation, which as well have undergone clonal propagation, enter the memory B-cell pool again. Due to high rates of division in clonal propagation and because EBV seems to increase genomic instability [91], there might be, although very rarely but more frequently than without EBV, *c-myc* translocations which lead to uncontrolled growth and tumour formation characteristic for BL. Moreover, a recent publication describes activated memory B-cells in GC reactions which undergo a second clonal propagation and somatic hypermutation for even higher affinity, which further increases the probability of accumulating transforming genetic hits [99]. To assign possible functions of LMP2B depending on B-cell differentiation stage in our model, we hypothesize that expression of LMP2B in activated memory B-cells might lead to decreased LMP2A activity and increased Scr levels (Figure 2B). The restoration of proper BCR signalling forces the activated memory B-cell towards a plasma cell phenotype and disrupts latent EBV infection.

6. XBP-1: cellular sensor for latent EBV disruption

Recent publications identified the host cell gene X-box binding protein (XBP)-1 as a factor responsible for the termination of latent EBV infection [6, 7]. XBP-1 is a leucin zipper transcriptional activator protein, which is upregulated in the early processes of terminal plasma cell differentiation. It belongs to the CREB/ATF family and upregulates the transcription of the master EBV lytic regulator gene *BZLF1*. Whether XBP-1 interacts directly with the promoter region of *BZLF1* or exploits an indirect pathway remains controversial [6, 7]. Importantly, Bhende et al. [7] and Sun et al. [6] reported lytic EBV infection upon XBP-1 activation. These findings are supported by the identification of lytic EBV infection in plasma cells of tonsillar B-cells *in vivo* [97, 100] and in tonsillar B-cells infected with EBV *ex vivo* undergoing terminal differentiation (Dorner et al., accepted for publication in JVI). Furthermore, it was shown that Kaposi's sarcoma-associated herpesviruses (KSHV) are activated by XBP-1 or that human CMV [101] and HTLV-1 [102] use XBP-1 in their life cycle.

Thus, EBV terminates its latent infection by hijacking the XBP-1 pathway. This enables the virus not only to use the enhanced transcription and translation machinery from the differentiating plasma cell but serves as well as back door for the virus to escape the host cell doomed to death due to terminal differentiation. On the other hand, as EBV is found preferentially *in vivo* in its latent form, the virus might have evolved effective mechanisms to regulate or even suppress its activation. Therefore, the upregulation of viral genes hijacking and blocking the terminal plasma cell differentiation process would allow the maintenance of persistence. As the physiological plasma cell differentiation, which includes the upregulation of plasma cell-specific transcription factors like BLIMP-1, XBP-1, and the unfolded protein response (UPR) [95-98], takes several days, there might be enough time for this intervention. Such a viral gene interfering with the plasma cell differentiation inducing signal is, as described above, LMLP2A.

Concluding remarks

In summary, recent publications hint to the existence of viral and cellular sensors in the regulation of latent and lytic EBV infection. LMP2B seems to regulate the dual function of LMP2A comprised of BCR block and survival signal. These findings suggest a function of LMP2B acting as a rheostat of LMP2A signal strength in B cells. The fact that LMP2B is conserved in EBV over the evolution and shares sequence homologies even with the rhesus monkey lymphocryptovirus (LCV) infecting Old World primates [103], indicate a strong selective pressure and an important function of LMP2B in the regulation of latent and lytic EBV infection. On the other hand, XBP-1 seems to be involved directly in the termination of latent EBV infection and links it to plasma cell differentiation. To amalgate the roles of LMP2B and XBP-1 in terminating latent EBV infection, will be an issue of future research. It might be that LMP2B acts on transcriptional and/or translational level on XBP-1 and vice versa. Additionally, there might as well be factors which drive the expression of LMP2B or stabilize the protein. However, which cellular factors these are and if they are dependent only on the plasma cell differentiation stage or on other factors as well, like senescence or stress, remains elusive and needs further investigations.

Acknowledgements

We would like to thank Marcus Dorner and Jürg Sigrist for fruitful discussion.

References

1. Thorley-Lawson, D.A. (2001) Epstein-Barr virus: exploiting the immune system. *Nat Rev Immunol* 1, 75-82
2. Longnecker, R. (2000) Epstein-Barr virus latency: LMP2, a regulator or means for Epstein-Barr virus persistence? *Adv Cancer Res* 79, 175-200
3. Rechsteiner, M.P., et al. (2007) Silencing of latent membrane protein 2B reduces susceptibility to activation of lytic Epstein-Barr virus in Burkitt's lymphoma Akata cells. *J Gen Virol* 88, 1454-1459
4. Rechsteiner, M.P., et al. (2007) Latent Membrane Protein 2B Regulates Susceptibility to Induction of Lytic Epstein-Barr Virus Infection. *J Virol*
5. Rovedo, M., and Longnecker, R. (2007) Epstein-barr virus latent membrane protein 2B (LMP2B) modulates LMP2A activity. *J Virol* 81, 84-94
6. Sun, C.C., and Thorley-Lawson, D.A. (2007) Plasma cell-specific transcription factor XBP-1s binds to and transactivates the Epstein-Barr virus BZLF1 promoter. *J Virol* 81, 13566-13577
7. Bhende, P.M., et al. (2007) X-box-binding protein 1 activates lytic Epstein-Barr virus gene expression in combination with protein kinase D. *J Virol* 81, 7363-7370
8. Murray, P.G., and Young, L.S. (2002) The Role of the Epstein-Barr virus in human disease. *Frontiers in Bioscience* 7, d519-540
9. Young, L.S., and Murray, P.G. (2003) Epstein-Barr virus and oncogenesis: from latent genes to tumours. *Oncogene* 22, 5108-5121
10. Rickinson, A., and Kieff, E. (2001) Epstein-Barr Virus. In *Fields Virology* (4th edn) (Knipe, D.M., and Howley, P.M., eds), 2575-2627, Lippincott Williams & Wilkins Publishers
11. Freemann, W.H. (2000) Kuby Immunology. *Fourth edition*
12. Laux, G., et al. (1989) The terminal protein gene 2 of Epstein-Barr virus is transcribed from a bidirectional latent promoter region. *J. Gen. Virol.* 70, 3079-3084
13. Laux, G., et al. (1988) A spliced Epstein-Barr virus gene expressed in immortalized lymphocytes is created by circularization of the linear viral genome. *EMBO J.* 7, 769-774
14. Sample, J., et al. (1989) Two related Epstein-Barr virus membrane proteins are encoded by separate genes. *J. Virol.* 63, 933-937

15. Brinkmann, M.M., and Schulz, T.F. (2006) Regulation of intracellular signalling by the terminal membrane proteins of members of the Gammaherpesvirinae. *J Gen Virol* 87, 1047-1074
16. Matskova, L., et al. (2001) C-terminal domain of the Epstein-Barr virus LMP2A membrane protein contains a clustering signal. *J Virol* 75, 10941-10949
17. Thompson, M.P., and Kurzrock, R. (2004) Epstein-Barr virus and cancer. *Clin Cancer Res* 10, 803-821
18. Cesarman, E. (2002) Epstein-Barr virus (EBV) and lymphomagenesis. *Frontiers in Bioscience* 7, e58-65
19. Rickinson, A.B., Kieff, E. (2007) Epstein-Barr Virus and its Replication
    In: David, P.M.H, Knipe, M. (Eds.), Fields Virology, vol. II. Lippincott-Raven Publishers, Philadelphia, Pa (Section II 68B)
20. Thorley-Lawson, D.A. (2005) EBV the prototypical human tumor virus--just how bad is it? *J Allergy Clin Immunol* 116, 251-261; quiz 262
21. Thorley-Lawson, D.A., and Gross, A. (2004) Persistence of the Epstein-Barr virus and the origins of associated lymphomas. *N Engl J Med* 350, 1328-1337
22. Babcock, G.J., and Thorley-Lawson, D.A. (2000) Tonsillar memory B cells, latently infected with Epstein-Barr virus, express the restricted pattern of latent genes previously found only in Epstein-Barr virus-associated tumors. *Proc Natl Acad Sci U S A* 97, 12250-12255
23. Ben-Sasson, S.A., and Klein, G. (1981) Activation of the Epstein-Barr virus genome by 5-aza-cytidine in latently infected human lymphoid lines. *Int J Cancer* 28, 131-135
24. Ernberg, I., et al. (1989) The role of methylation in the phenotype-dependent modulation of Epstein-Barr nuclear antigen 2 and latent membrane protein genes in cells latently infected with Epstein-Barr virus. *J Gen Virol* 70, 2989-3002
25. Jansson, A., et al. (1992) Methylation of discrete sites within the enhancer region regulates the activity of the Epstein-Barr virus BamHI W promoter in Burkitt lymphoma lines. *J Virol* 66, 62-69
26. Masucci, M.G., et al. (1989) 5-Azacytidine up regulates the expression of Epstein-Barr virus nuclear antigen 2 (EBNA-2) through EBNA-6 and latent membrane protein in the Burkitt's lymphoma line rael. *J Virol* 63, 3135-3141
27. Rao, S.P., et al. (2007) Zebularine reactivates silenced E-cadherin but unlike 5-Azacytidine does not induce switching from latent to lytic Epstein-Barr virus infection in Burkitt's lymphoma Akata cells. *Mol Cancer* 6, 3

28. Kelly, K., and Knox, K.A. (1995) Differential regulatory effects of cAMP-elevating agents on human normal and neoplastic B cell functional response following ligation of surface immunoglobulin and CD40. *Cell Immunol* 166, 93-102
29. di Renzo, L., *et al.* (1994) Endogenous TGF-beta contributes to the induction of the EBV lytic cycle in two Burkitt lymphoma cell lines. *Int J Cancer* 57, 914-919
30. Casola, S., *et al.* (2004) B cell receptor signal strength determines B cell fate. *Nat Immunol* 5, 317-327
31. Caldwell, R.G., *et al.* (2000) Epstein-Barr virus LMP2A-induced B-cell survival in two unique classes of EmuLMP2A transgenic mice. *J Virol* 74, 1101-1113
32. Ikeda, A., *et al.* (2003) Itchy, a Nedd4 ubiquitin ligase, downregulates latent membrane protein 2A activity in B-cell signaling. *J Virol* 77, 5529-5534
33. Ikeda, A., *et al.* (2004) Latent membrane protein 2A, a viral B cell receptor homologue, induces CD5+ B-1 cell development. *J Immunol* 172, 5329-5337
34. Portis, T., *et al.* (2004) Epstein-Barr virus LMP2A: regulating cellular ubiquitination processes for maintenance of viral latency? *Trends Immunol* 25, 422-426
35. Merchant, M., *et al.* (2000) The LMP2A ITAM is essential for providing B cells with development and survival signals in vivo. *J Virol* 74, 9115-9124
36. Osborne, B., and Miele, L. (1999) Notch and the immune system. *Immunity* 11, 653-663
37. Takasawa, M., *et al.* (2002) Automatic determination of brain perfusion index for measurement of cerebral blood flow using spectral analysis and 99mTc-HMPAO. *Eur J Nucl Med Mol Imaging* 29, 1443-1446
38. Maillard, I., *et al.* (2003) Notch and the immune system. *Immunity* 19, 781-791
39. Jundt, F., *et al.* (2002) Activated Notch1 signaling promotes tumor cell proliferation and survival in Hodgkin and anaplastic large cell lymphoma. *Blood* 99, 3398-3403
40. Anderson, L.J., and Longnecker, R. (2007) An auto-regulatory loop for EBV LMP2A involves activation of Notch. *Virology*
41. Allen, M.D., *et al.* (2005) The Epstein-Barr virus-encoded LMP2A and LMP2B proteins promote epithelial cell spreading and motility. *J Virol* 79, 1789-1802
42. Fruehling, S., *et al.* (1996) Identification of latent membrane protein 2A (LMP2A) domains essential for the LMP2A dominant-negative effect on B-lymphocyte surface immunoglobulin signal transduction. *J Virol* 70, 6216-6226
43. Ikeda, M., and Longnecker, R. (2007) Cholesterol is critical for Epstein-Barr virus latent membrane protein 2A trafficking and protein stability. *Virology* 360, 461-468

44. Longnecker, R., et al. (1991) An Epstein-Barr virus protein associated with cell growth transformation interacts with a tyrosine kinase. *J Virol* 65, 3681-3692
45. Longnecker, R., and Kieff, E. (1990) A second Epstein-Barr virus membrane protein (LMP2) is expressed in latent infection and colocalizes with LMP1. *J Virol* 64, 2319-2326
46. Lynch, D.T., et al. (2002) Epstein-Barr virus latent membrane protein 2B (LMP2B) co-localizes with LMP2A in perinuclear regions in transiently transfected cells. *J Gen Virol* 83, 1025-1035
47. Tomaszewski-Flick, M.J., and Rowe, D.T. (2007) Minimal protein domain requirements for the intracellular localization and self-aggregation of Epstein-Barr Virus Latent Membrane Protein 2. *Virus Genes* 35, 225-234
48. Heussinger, N., et al. (2004) Expression of the Epstein-Barr virus (EBV)-encoded latent membrane protein 2A (LMP2A) in EBV-associated nasopharyngeal carcinoma. *J Pathol* 203, 696-699
49. Portis, T., et al. (2002) The LMP2A signalosome--a therapeutic target for Epstein-Barr virus latency and associated disease. *Front Biosci* 7, d414-426
50. Higuchi, M., et al. (2001) Epstein-Barr virus latent-infection membrane proteins are palmitoylated and raft-associated: protein 1 binds to the cytoskeleton through TNF receptor cytoplasmic factors. *Proc Natl Acad Sci U S A* 98, 4675-4680
51. Katzman, R.B., and Longnecker, R. (2004) LMP2A does not require palmitoylation to localize to buoyant complexes or for function. *J Virol* 78, 10878-10887
52. Ikeda, M., Fukuda, M., Longnecker, R. (2005) Epstein-Barr Virus. Function of Latent Membrane Protein 2A. *Caister Academic Press*
53. Ikeda, M., et al. (2000) The Epstein-Barr virus latent membrane protein 2A PY motif recruits WW domain-containing ubiquitin-protein ligases. *Virology* 268, 178-191
54. Winberg, G., et al. (2000) Latent membrane protein 2A of Epstein-Barr virus binds WW domain E3 protein-ubiquitin ligases that ubiquitinate B-cell tyrosine kinases. *Mol Cell Biol* 20, 8526-8535
55. Hicke, L. (2001) A new ticket for entry into budding vesicles-ubiquitin. *Cell* 106, 527-530
56. Wilkinson, K.D. (2000) Ubiquitination and deubiquitination: targeting of proteins for degradation by the proteasome. *Semin Cell Dev Biol* 11, 141-148
57. Rechsteiner, M.P., et al. (2008) Latent membrane protein 2B regulates susceptibility to induction of lytic Epstein-Barr virus infection. *J Virol* 82, 1739-1747

58. Cohen, J.I. (2000) Epstein-Barr virus infection. *N Engl J Med* 343, 481-492
59. Wang, X., and Hutt-Fletcher, L.M. (1998) Epstein-Barr virus lacking glycoprotein gp42 can bind to B cells but is not able to infect. *J Virol* 72, 158-163
60. Wang, X., *et al.* (1998) Epstein-Barr virus uses different complexes of glycoproteins gH and gL to infect B lymphocytes and epithelial cells. *J Virol* 72, 5552-5558
61. Khanna, R., *et al.* (1999) Vaccine strategies against Epstein-Barr virus-associated diseases: lessons from studies on cytotoxic T-cell-mediated immune regulation. *Immunol Rev* 170, 49-64
62. Hochberg, D., *et al.* (2004) Demonstration of the Burkitt's lymphoma Epstein-Barr virus phenotype in dividing latently infected memory cells in vivo. *Proc Natl Acad Sci U S A* 101, 239-244
63. Souza, T.A., *et al.* (2007) Influence of EBV on the peripheral blood memory B cell compartment. *J Immunol* 179, 3153-3160
64. Kuppers, R. (2005) Mechanisms of B-cell lymphoma pathogenesis. *Nat Rev Cancer* 5, 251-262
65. Brauninger, A., *et al.* (2006) Molecular biology of Hodgkin's and Reed/Sternberg cells in Hodgkin's lymphoma. *Int J Cancer* 118, 1853-1861
66. Mancao, C., *et al.* (2005) Rescue of "crippled" germinal center B cells from apoptosis by Epstein-Barr virus. *Blood* 106, 4339-4344
67. Caldwell, R.G., *et al.* (1998) Epstein-Barr virus LMP2A drives B cell development and survival in the absence of normal B cell receptor signals. *Immunity* 9, 405-411
68. Swanson-Mungerson, M., *et al.* (2006) Epstein-Barr virus LMP2A enhances B-cell responses in vivo and in vitro. *J Virol* 80, 6764-6770
69. Swanson-Mungerson, M.A., *et al.* (2005) Epstein-Barr virus LMP2A alters in vivo and in vitro models of B-cell anergy, but not deletion, in response to autoantigen. *J Virol* 79, 7355-7362
70. Kurth, J., *et al.* (2000) EBV-infected B cells in infectious mononucleosis: viral strategies for spreading in the B cell compartment and establishing latency. *Immunity* 13, 485-495
71. Kurth, J., *et al.* (2003) Epstein-Barr virus-infected B cells expanding in germinal centers of infectious mononucleosis patients do not participate in the germinal center reaction. *Proc Natl Acad Sci U S A* 100, 4730-4735

72. Lee, J., et al. (2007) Effect of positive bone marrow EBV in situ hybridization in staging and survival of localized extranodal natural killer/T-cell lymphoma, nasal-type. Clin Cancer Res 13, 3250-3254
73. Kuppers, R., et al. (2002) Biology of Hodgkin's lymphoma. Ann Oncol 13 Suppl 1, 11-18
74. Portis, T., et al. (2003) Epstein-Barr Virus (EBV) LMP2A induces alterations in gene transcription similar to those observed in Reed-Sternberg cells of Hodgkin lymphoma. Blood 102, 4166-4178
75. Portis, T., and Longnecker, R. (2003) Epstein-Barr virus LMP2A interferes with global transcription factor regulation when expressed during B-lymphocyte development. J Virol 77, 105-114
76. Brooks, L., et al. (1992) Epstein-Barr virus latent gene transcription in nasopharyngeal carcinoma cells: coexpression of EBNA1, LMP1, and LMP2 transcripts. J Virol 66, 2689-2697
77. Busson, P., et al. (1995) Sequence polymorphism in the Epstein-Barr virus latent membrane protein (LMP)-2 gene. J Gen Virol 76 (Pt 1), 139-145
78. Niedobitek, G., et al. (1997) Immunohistochemical detection of the Epstein-Barr virus-encoded latent membrane protein 2A in Hodgkin's disease and infectious mononucleosis. Blood 90, 1664-1672
79. Ikeda, M., et al. (2001) PY motifs of Epstein-Barr virus LMP2A regulate protein stability and phosphorylation of LMP2A-associated proteins. J Virol 75, 5711-5718
80. Hardy, R.R., and Hayakawa, K. (2001) B cell development pathways. Annu Rev Immunol 19, 595-621
81. Swanson-Mungerson, M., and Longnecker, R. (2007) Epstein-Barr virus latent membrane protein 2A and autoimmunity. Trends Immunol 28, 213-218
82. Tosato, G., et al. (1984) Abnormally elevated frequency of Epstein-Barr virus-infected B cells in the blood of patients with rheumatoid arthritis. J Clin Invest 73, 1789-1795
83. James, J.A., et al. (2001) Systemic lupus erythematosus in adults is associated with previous Epstein-Barr virus exposure. Arthritis Rheum 44, 1122-1126
84. Haahr, S., and Hollsberg, P. (2006) Multiple sclerosis is linked to Epstein-Barr virus infection. Rev Med Virol 16, 297-310
85. Gross, A.J., et al. (2005) EBV and systemic lupus erythematosus: a new perspective. J Immunol 174, 6599-6607

86. Kuppers, R. (2003) B cells under influence: transformation of B cells by Epstein-Barr virus. *Nat Rev Immunol* 3, 801-812
87. Kieff, E., Rickinson, A.B. (2007) Epstein-Barr Virus and its Replication. *In: David, P.M.H, Knipe, M. (Eds.), Fields Virology, vol. II. Lippincott-Raven Publishers, Philadelphia, Pa (Section II 68A)*
88. Babcock, G.J., et al. (2000) The expression pattern of Epstein-Barr virus latent genes in vivo is dependent upon the differentiation stage of the infected B cell. *Immunity* 13, 497-506
89. Miller, C.L., et al. (1993) Epstein-Barr virus latent membrane protein 2A blocks calcium mobilization in B lymphocytes. *J Virol* 67, 3087-3094
90. Takada, K. (1984) Cross-linking of cell surface immunoglobulins induces Epstein-Barr virus in Burkitt lymphoma lines. *Int J Cancer* 33, 27-32
91. Kamranvar, S.A., et al. (2007) Epstein-Barr virus promotes genomic instability in Burkitt's lymphoma. *Oncogene* 26, 5115-5123
92. Bernasconi, M., et al. (2006) Quantitative profiling of housekeeping and Epstein-Barr virus gene transcription in Burkitt lymphoma cell lines using an oligonucleotide microarray. *Virol J* 3, 43
93. Yuan, J., et al. (2006) Virus and cell RNAs expressed during Epstein-Barr virus replication. *J Virol* 80, 2548-2565
94. Hadinoto, V., et al. (2008) On the dynamics of acute EBV infection and the pathogenesis of infectious mononucleosis. *Blood* 111, 1420-1427
95. Gass, J.N., et al. (2002) Activation of an unfolded protein response during differentiation of antibody-secreting B cells. *J Biol Chem* 277, 49047-49054
96. Arpin, C., et al. (1997) Memory B cells are biased towards terminal differentiation: a strategy that may prevent repertoire freezing. *J Exp Med* 186, 931-940
97. Laichalk, L.L., and Thorley-Lawson, D.A. (2005) Terminal differentiation into plasma cells initiates the replicative cycle of Epstein-Barr virus in vivo. *J Virol* 79, 1296-1307
98. Schroder, M., and Kaufman, R.J. (2005) The mammalian unfolded protein response. *Annu Rev Biochem* 74, 739-789
99. Bende, R.J., et al. (2007) Germinal centers in human lymph nodes contain reactivated memory B cells. *J Exp Med* 204, 2655-2665
100. Laichalk, L.L., et al. (2002) The dispersal of mucosal memory B cells: evidence from persistent EBV infection. *Immunity* 16, 745-754

101. Isler, J.A., *et al.* (2005) Human cytomegalovirus infection activates and regulates the unfolded protein response. *J Virol* 79, 6890-6899
102. Ku, S.C., *et al.* (2008) XBP-1, a novel HTLV-1 Tax binding protein, activates HTLV-1 basal and Tax-activated transcription. *J Virol*
103. Rivailler, P., *et al.* (1999) Strong selective pressure for evolution of an Epstein-Barr virus LMP2B homologue in the rhesus lymphocryptovirus. *J Virol* 73, 8867-8872

Figure legends

Figure1: Possible pathways how LMP2B might act as a rheostat for LMP2A and BCR signalling. *Left side panel*: Newly translated LMP2A dimerize in the TGN or in vesicles on the way to the plasma membrane. As there are no or only small amounts of Scr kinases and ubiquitin ligases present, LMP2A is able to reach the plasma membrane. Once arrived at the plasma membrane, LMP2A dimers are organized in a signalosome consisting of Scr kinases and ubiquitin ligases, leading to ubiquitination and internalization. Further polyubiquitination leads to degradation in proteasomes which results in a block of BCR signal once a specific antigen is encountered due to depletion of signalling proteins. Another possible pathway might exist in the fusion of the endocytosed signalosome with a LMP2B containing vesicle. LMP2B is able to disrupt LMP2A homodimers which induces deubiquitination by deubiquitinating enzymes (DUBs). Deubiquitination allows a turn-over of internalized proteins back to the cell surface and restores proper BCR signalling. *Middle panel*: LMP2B and LMP2A heterodimers segregate to the plasma membrane. As there is no activation of LMP2A, enough Scr kinases are present in the case of a BCR signal induced from an antigen. At the plasma membrane there might occur disassembly and reassembly of either LMP2A (described above) or LMP2B (described below) homodimers depending on the expression levels of both proteins. *Right side panel*: LMP2B homodimers on the plasma membrane would allow an intact BCR signal upon antigen encounter.

Figure2: Effects of LMP2B and LMP2A on B-cell differentiation. (A) *Germinal centre:* Non-functional class switch or hypermutation normally leads to cell death. EBV rescues these B cells by the expression of LMP2A. These surviving B cells might give rise to the formation of HL. Hypermutation generates (i) low and (ii) high affinity B cells for foreign antigens. (i) LMP2A and low BCR signal together might result in strong enough signal for proper germinal centre (GC) reaction and differentiation into a memory B-cell. (ii) LMP2B might abolish the activity of LMP2A, thus enabling proper BCR signal. The GC reaction favours, among others, c-myc translocation and p53 malfunction, increasing the possibility of Burkitt's lymphoma (BL) formation. (B) *Blood and secondary lymphoid tissue:* Upon foreign antigen encounter, a specific memory B-cell is activated and starts with clonal expansion. A part of the cells expands for the maintenance of the memory B-cell pool. Another part starts to differentiate into plasma cells. As EBV tries to maintain latency, it upregulates LMP2A, in that way blocking BCR signalling and lytic EBV activation. Increased division in clonal propagation favours *c-myc* translocation and p53 malfunction which may lead to the formation of BL. LMP2B might be stabilized by yet unknown factors in the cells (i.e. plasma cell factors, senescence, stress). LMP2B disrupts the ability of LMP2A to block BCR signalling and forces the memory B-cell towards plasma cell fate. XBP-1 is upregulated in terminal plasma cell differentiation and triggers lytic EBV.

Figure 1: Possible pathways how LMP2B might act as a rheostat for LMP2A and BCR signalling

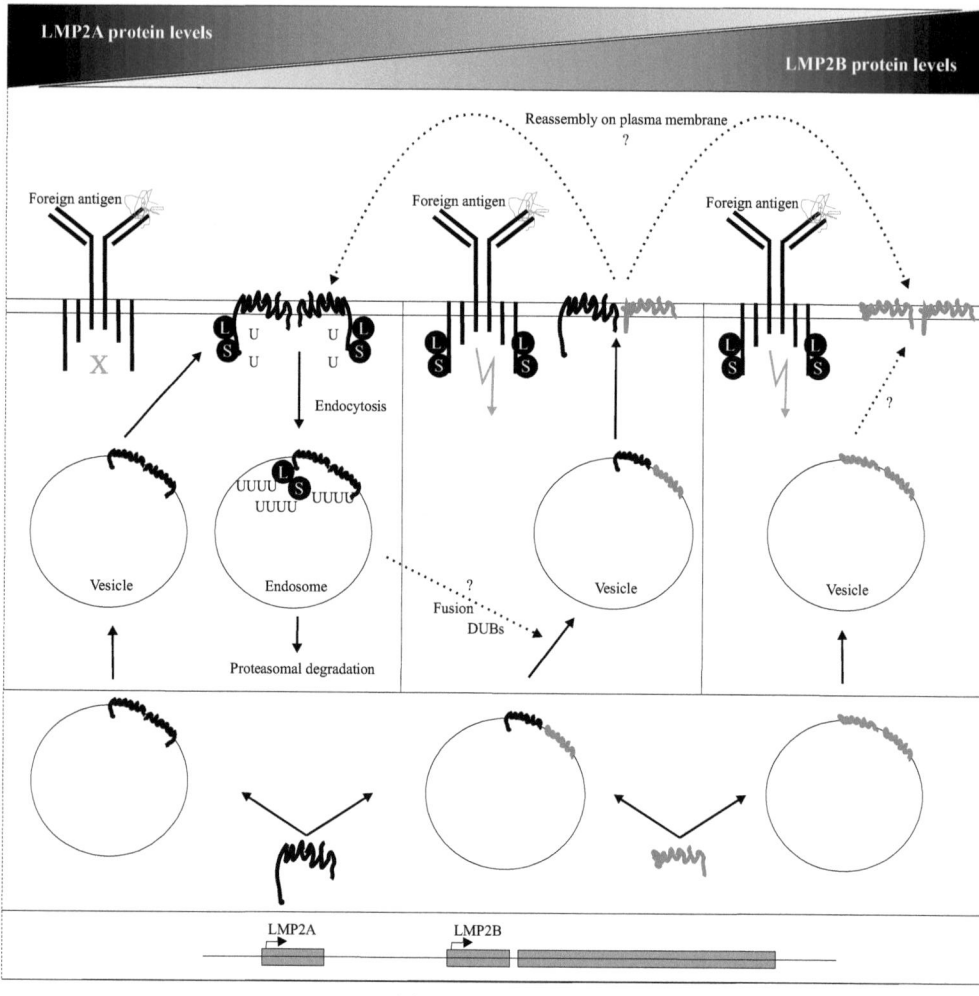

Figure 2: Effects of LMP2B and LMP2A on B-cell differentiation

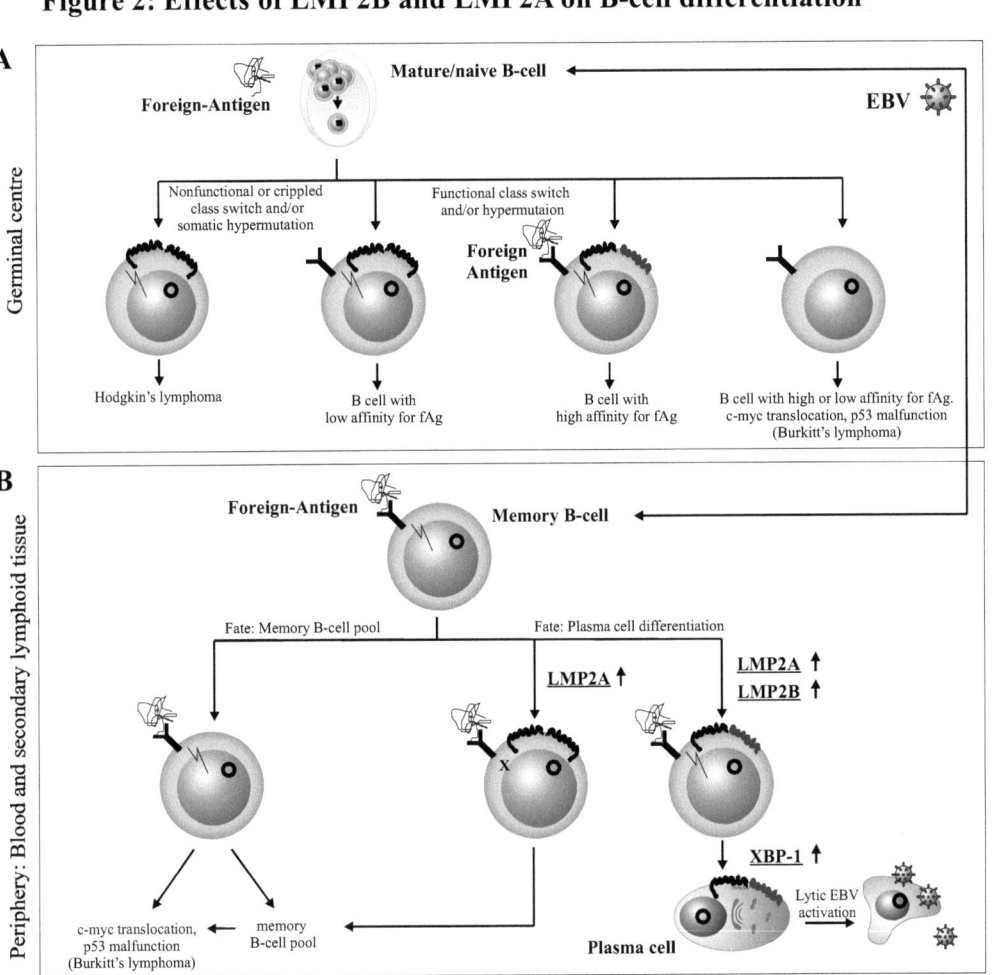

5. Subject of investigation

Due to the fact, that EBV-associated malignancies are treated nowadays with radio- and chemotherapy with still not satisfactory cure rates including severe side effects and due to the fact, that these tumors contain EBV in up to 100% of the tumor mass, gave rise to the formulation of a new tumor therapy: <u>induction of lytic EBV infection leading to destruction of EBV-harboring tumor cells</u>. Although EBV has been known for several decades, there are still many unknowns in the equation of how the virus regulates its latent and lytic form. Thus, the aim of this thesis was to determine factors destabilizing latent EBV infection. As a promising target, we selected the latent membrane protein (LMP)2B, about which we got evidence in preliminary studies to increase lytic EBV infection upon activation of the virus harboring B-cell. To elucidate the mechanism how LMP2B may be involved in the regulation of lytic EBV infection, we approached the question on the one hand by silencing LMP2B and on the other hand by overexpression. As a system to study the impact of silencing and overexpression of LMP2B we chose the EBV positive BL cell line Akata in which lytic EBV infection can be triggered using BCR cross-linking.

Our concept of exploiting switching from latent EBV infection to lytic infection could as well serve as a model to fight other herpes viral-induced cancers. Finally, this project could also lead to new insights assisting the improvement of silencing or overexpression of genes from other viruses contributing to cancer development as , e.g., HCV or, more generally, of human oncogenes. The ultimate goal is the translation of these experimental efforts to the bedside, for treatment of patients affected by malignancies associated with EBV.

6. Results

6.1 Zebularine reactivates silenced E-cadherin but unlike 5-Azacytidine does not induce switching from latent to lytic Epstein-Barr virus infection in Burkitt lymphoma Akata cells.
Rao SP, Rechsteiner MP, Berger C, Sigrist JA, Nadal D, Bernasconi M., Molecular Cancer, **6**:3 (2007).

Abstract

Epigenetic silencing of regulatory genes by aberrant methylation contributes to tumorigenesis. DNA methyltransferase inhibitors (DNMTI) represent promising new drugs for anti-cancer therapies. The DNMTI 5-Azacytidine is effective against myelodysplastic syndrome, but induces switching of latent to lytic Epstein-Barr virus (EBV) in vitro and results in EBV DNA demethylation with the potential of induction of lytic EBV in vivo. This is of considerable concern given that recurrent lytic EBV has been linked with an increased incidence of EBV-associated lymphomas. Based on the distinct properties of action we hypothesized that the newer DNMTI Zebularine might differ from 5-Azacytidine in its potential to induce switching from latent to lytic EBV. Here we show that both 5-Azacytidine and Zebularine are able to induce expression of E-cadherin, a cellular gene frequently silenced by hypermethylation in cancers, and thus demonstrate that both DNMTI are active in our experimental setting consisting of EBV-harboring Burkitt's lymphoma Akata cells. Quantification of mRNA expression of EBV genes revealed that 5-Azacytidine induces switching from latent to lytic EBV and, in addition, that the immediate-early lytic infection progresses to early and late lytic infection. Furthermore, 5-Azacytidine induced upregulation of the latent EBV genes LMP2A, LMP2B, and EBNA2 in a similar fashion as observed following switching of latent to lytic EBV upon cross-linking of the B-cell receptor. In striking contrast, Zebularine did not exhibit any effect neither on lytic nor on latent EBV gene expression. Thus, Zebularine might be safer than 5-Azacytidine for the treatment of cancers in EBV carriers and could also be applied against EBV-harboring tumors, since it does not induce switching from latent to lytic EBV which may result in secondary EBV-associated malignancies.

Molecular Cancer

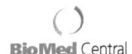

Short communication

Zebularine reactivates silenced *E-cadherin* but unlike 5-Azacytidine does not induce switching from latent to lytic Epstein-Barr virus infection in Burkitt's lymphoma Akata cells

Sieta P Rao, Markus P Rechsteiner, Christoph Berger, Jürg A Sigrist, David Nadal† and Michele Bernasconi*†

Address: Experimental Infectious Diseases and Cancer Research, University Children's Hospital, University of Zurich, August Forel Str. 1, CH-8008 Zürich, Switzerland
Email: Sieta P Rao - s.p.rao@access.unizh.ch; Markus P Rechsteiner - markus.rechsteiner@kispi.unizh.ch; Christoph Berger - christoph.berger@kispi.unizh.ch; Jürg A Sigrist - juerg.sigrist@kispi.unizh.ch; David Nadal - david.nadal@kispi.unizh.ch; Michele Bernasconi* - michele.bernasconi@kispi.unizh.ch
* Corresponding author   †Equal contributors

Published: 10 January 2007

Molecular Cancer 2007, **6**:3 doi:10.1186/1476-4598-6-3

Received: 24 November 2006
Accepted: 10 January 2007

This article is available from: http://www.molecular-cancer.com/content/6/1/3

© 2007 Rao et al; licensee BioMed Central Ltd.
This is an Open Access article distributed under the terms of the Creative Commons Attribution License (http://creativecommons.org/licenses/by/2.0), which permits unrestricted use, distribution, and reproduction in any medium, provided the original work is properly cited.

Abstract

Epigenetic silencing of regulatory genes by aberrant methylation contributes to tumorigenesis. DNA methyltransferase inhibitors (DNMTI) represent promising new drugs for anti-cancer therapies. The DNMTI 5-Azacytidine is effective against myelodysplastic syndrome, but induces switching of latent to lytic Epstein-Barr virus (EBV) *in vitro* and results in EBV DNA demethylation with the potential of induction of lytic EBV *in vivo*. This is of considerable concern given that recurrent lytic EBV has been linked with an increased incidence of EBV-associated lymphomas. Based on the distinct properties of action we hypothesized that the newer DNMTI Zebularine might differ from 5-Azacytidine in its potential to induce switching from latent to lytic EBV. Here we show that both 5-Azacytidine and Zebularine are able to induce expression of *E-cadherin*, a cellular gene frequently silenced by hypermethylation in cancers, and thus demonstrate that both DNMTI are active in our experimental setting consisting of EBV-harboring Burkitt's lymphoma Akata cells. Quantification of mRNA expression of EBV genes revealed that 5-Azacytidine induces switching from latent to lytic EBV and, in addition, that the immediate-early lytic infection progresses to early and late lytic infection. Furthermore, 5-Azacytidine induced upregulation of the latent EBV genes *LMP2A*, *LMP2B*, and *EBNA2* in a similar fashion as observed following switching of latent to lytic EBV upon cross-linking of the B-cell receptor. In striking contrast, Zebularine did not exhibit any effect neither on lytic nor on latent EBV gene expression. Thus, Zebularine might be safer than 5-Azacytidine for the treatment of cancers in EBV carriers and could also be applied against EBV-harboring tumors, since it does not induce switching from latent to lytic EBV which may result in secondary EBV-associated malignancies.

Findings

Abnormal hypermethylation of the promoters of cancer-related or tumor suppressor genes is commonly found in primary neoplasms and tumor cell lines [1]. Thus, pharmacologic inhibition of DNA methylation could provide an effective means of epigenetic anti-cancer treatment.

Indeed, 5-Azacytidine, a pyrimidine ring analogue of cytidine and DNA methylase inhibitor (DNMTI), has proven to be effective against myelodysplastic syndrome in a phase III randomized clinical trial [2]. 5-Azacytidine forms covalent complexes with cytosine- [C5]-specific DNA methyltransferases and inhibits their activity [3]. In addition, 5-Azacytidine is activated by uridine-cytidine kinase and can be incorporated into both RNA and DNA. Incorporation into RNA interferes with protein translation [4], which is the cause of 5-Azacytidine toxicity. This substance is also characterized by a low stability in aqueous solution [5,6].

Different types of cancers including Burkitt's lymphoma (BL) and nasopharyngeal carcinoma (NPC) harbor latent Epstein Barr virus (EBV) [7] and maintenance of latent EBV is partially mediated by hypermethylation of the EBV genome. Thus, it is not surprising that 5-Azacytidine induces switching of latent to lytic EBV in vitro [8-11] and results in EBV DNA demethylation in NPC patients with the potential of induction of lytic EBV [12]. Recurrent lytic EBV caused by chronic disruption of EBV latency due to long-lasting methotrexate treatment in EBV-carrying rheumatoid arthritis and polymyositis patients has been linked with an increased incidence of EBV-associated lymphomas [13]. Therefore, since DNMTI need to be administered for long periods of time to treat cancers, DNMTI with the potential to induce lytic EBV could have detrimental consequences in EBV carriers and be inappropriate to combat EBV-carrying tumors.

Zebularine (1-(β-D-ribofuranosyl)-1,2-dihydropyrimidin-2-one), a newer cytidine analog containing a 2-(1H)-pyrimidinone ring, acts as 5-Azacytidine by forming covalent complexes with DNMT [14], and in addition acts as transition state analog inhibitor of cytidine deaminase by binding covalently at the active site [15]. In comparison to 5-Azacytidine, Zebularine has little toxicity; shows increased stability [16,17], and targets preferentially tumor cells [18]. Hence, Zebularine promises to be a better drug than 5-Azacytidine for epigenetic therapy of cancer. Nevertheless, the potential of Zebularine in inducing lytic EBV is unknown.

Based on the distinct properties we hypothesized that Zebularine might differ from 5-Azacytidine in its potential to induce lytic EBV. Thus, we compared the effects of both DNMTI on EBV latency in the BL cell line Akata, a well-established model to study switching of latent to lytic EBV which also allows the study of DNMTI effects on cellular genes silenced in cancer cells.

We first determined the concentrations of 5-Azacytidine and Zebularine without cytotoxicity within 48 h. The highest sub-toxic concentration of 5-Azacytidine was 1 µM (Fig. 1a) and of Zebularine was between 0.03 mM and 0.1 mM (Fig. 1b).

To validate our experimental conditions we next measured in Akata cells the expression of cellular genes known to be reactivated by Zebularine in other tumor cell lines including CDKN1A, CDKN1B and CDKN2A genes [18,19]. Using quantitative real-time PCR (qRT-PCR), expression of these cyclin-dependent kinases (CDK) was already detectable in the non-treated cells and did not further increase upon treatment neither with 5-Azacytidine nor Zebularine (not shown) suggesting that in the p53 mutated Akata cells [20] these CDKs are not silenced by hypermethylation. This did not hold true for E-cadherin (CDH1). E-cadherin mediates cell adhesion and loss of its expression by hypermethylation [21] is responsible for increased cancer invasiveness and metastasis [22]. CDH1 expression is reactivated by 5-aza-2'-deoxycytidine treatment in the BL cell line Raji [23]. We therefore measured the expression of CDH1 by qRT-PCR in treated Akata cells (Fig. 1c and 1d). Expression of CDH1 was not detectable in non-treated Akata cells. Treatment with 1.0 µM 5-Azacytidine resulted in a 30-fold induction of CDH1 mRNA expression after 48 h, that increased to 150-fold at 72 h. At a concentration of 0.5 µM, 5-Azacytidine showed a maximal 30-fold activation of CDH1 after 72 h and at 0.1 µM had no significant effect on expression of CDH1 mRNA even after 72 h. Zebularine (100 µM) induced a 50-fold activation of CDH1 after 120 h (5 days), that was sustained and increased to 100-fold after 10 days of continuous Zebularine treatment. This delayed effect was expected since Zebularine follows a slower kinetic with maximal effects later than 5-Azacytidine also in other cellular backgrounds [18,24]. These results show that 5-Azacytidine and Zebularine are able to induce expression of CDH1 known to be frequently silenced by hypermethylation [22,25], and demonstrate that both DNMTI are active in our experimental setting.

The first step in activation of lytic EBV infection is the expression of the immediate-early lytic EBV gene BZLF1. Zta, the product of BZLF1, is a transcription factor that regulates the expression of early lytic EBV genes, and activates the lytic EBV gene expression program [26]. To determine the effects of 5-Azacytidine and Zebularine on switching latent to lytic EBV in Akata cells, we measured the mRNA expression of BZLF1 by qRT-PCR in Akata cells treated with increasing concentrations of 5-Azacytidine at 48 h and 72 h and for Zebularine at up to 10 days. 1 µM 5-Azacytidine was able to induce activation of BZLF1 mRNA expression (Fig 1e). Induction of BZLF1 mRNA was robust, reaching about 280-fold over mock-treated cells. 5-Azacytidine concentrations lower than 1 µM did not have a significant effect on BZLF1 mRNA expression. Cytotoxic concentrations higher than 1 µM also activated

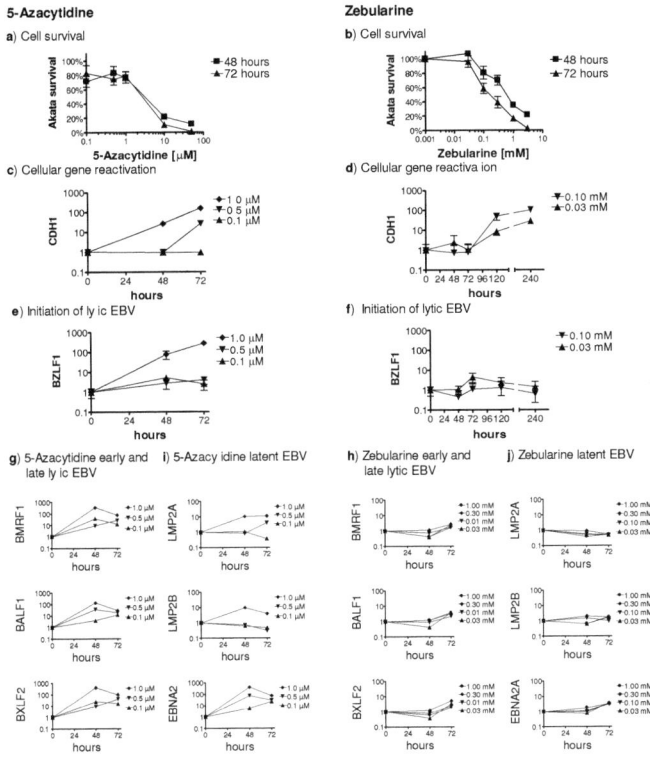

Figure 1
Response of Burkitt's lymphoma Akata cells to 5-Azacytidine and Zebularine treatment. **(a, b) Determination of non-toxic concentrations for Akata treatment** *in vitro* with 5-Azacytidine (a) and Zebularine (b). 5 × 10⁵ viable cells were seeded in 1 ml medium with increasing 5-Azacytidine or Zebularine concentrations. Living cells (trypan-blue exclusion) were then counted after 48 h and 72 h. The highest non-toxic-concentrations are: 1 μM 5-Azacytidine (a) and 100 μM for Zebularine (b). **(c, d) Expression of E-cadherin (CDH1)** normalized to *HMBS*. Treatment with 1.0 μM 5-Azacytidine resulted in a 30-fold induction of *CDH1* expression after 48 h (c), and with slower kinetics 100 μM Zebularine induced a 60-fold activation after 120 h and was sustained after 8 days of continuous Zebularine treatment (d). **(e, f) BZLF1 expression** indicating initiation of lytic EBV was observed after 1 μM 5-Azacytidine treatment (e), while 30 μM or 100 μM Zebularine do not activate *BZLF1* expression, even after 8 days (f). Data in a-f are given as means ± SD from three independent experiments **(g, h) Expression of early and late lytic EBV genes**. Treatment with 5-Azacytidine results in increased expression of both EBV early and late antigens (g). Treatment with Zebularine did not show any significant increase of expression of early or late lytic antigens (h). **(i, j) Expression of latent EBV genes** *LMP2A* and *EBNA2* increased around 10-fold upon treatment with 1.0 μM 5-Azacytidine. *EBNA2* expression increased about 60-fold by 0.5 μM and 1.0 μM 5-Azacytidine at 48 h. The lowest 5-Azacytidine concentration used (0.1 μM) was also able to induce a 50-fold increase of *EBNA2* expression at 72 h (i). *LMP2B* did show a maximal increase when treated with 1 μM 5-Azacytidine. (i). Treatment with Zebularine concentrations between 0.03 mM and 1 mM did not have a significant effect on *LMP2B* and *EBNA2* gene expression up to 72 h (j). Data in g-j are given as means of three independent experiments.

BZLF1 mRNA expression to even a greater extent (not shown). Treatment of Akata cells with 100 µM Zebularine did not result in induction of BZLF1 mRNA (Fig. 1f). Higher concentrations of Zebularine in the range of 1 mM to 3 mM resulted in a 10-fold induction of BZLF1 mRNA (not shown), likely due to stress response to cytotoxic insult, rather than specific activation of BZLF1 mRNA expression. These results confirm that 5-Azacytidine initiates lytic EBV infection at sub-toxic concentrations and in addition demonstrate that by contrast treatment with Zebularine up to 10 days does not provoke any change in BZLF1 mRNA expression levels in Akata cells.

To elucidate whether activation of the master regulatory lytic EBV gene BZLF1 by 5-Azacytidine is followed by activation of early and late lytic EBV genes and whether Zebularine does activate other lytic EBV genes independently of BZLF1 we also quantified mRNA expression of BALF1, BMRF1, and BXLF2 (Fig. 1g and 1h). BALF1 codes for an anti-apoptotic cytoplasmic early lytic antigen, BMRF1 for the early antigen-diffuse EA-D, and BXLF2 for the late lytic antigen glycoprotein gp85. Treatment of Akata cells with 1 µM 5-Azacytidine resulted in increased expression of both early and the late lytic antigens at 48 h with surprisingly similar kinetics. Even 0.1 µM 5-Azacytidine was able to increase mRNA expression of lytic EBV genes by a tenfold at 72 h. By contrast, no expression of early or late lytic EBV genes was measurable in Akata cells treated with Zebularine. Even treatment with 1 mM Zebularine; a concentration that apparently did induce expression of BZLF1 mRNA after 48 h, was not able to activate mRNA expression of other lytic EBV genes. This supports our above mentioned interpretation that expression of BZLF1 mRNA at a 1 mM Zebularine dose was not a specific event with subsequent full lytic EBV gene expression. These results indicate that 5-Azacytidine activates all three phases of lytic EBV infection and evidence that Zebularine does not induce switching from latent to lytic EBV.

The failure of Zebularine to induce switching from latent to lytic EBV could be due to either having no effect on EBV at all or due to reinforcement of latent EBV gene expression. Thus, we compared the quantitative mRNA expression of latent EBV genes before and during treatment with 5-Azacytidine or Zebularine. Treatment of Akata cells with 1.0 µM and 0.5 µM 5-Azacytidine increased LMP2A mRNA expression by 10-fold at 48 h and at 72 h, respectively, and LMP2B mRNA by around 10-fold at 48 h (1.0 µM). The effects on EBNA2 mRNA expression were more marked with an increase by 60-fold using 5-Azacytidine at 0.5 µM and by 400-fold at 1.0 µM at 48 h. Even the lowest 5-Azacytidine concentration used (0.1 µM) was able to induce a 30-fold increase of EBNA2 mRNA expression at 72 h (Fig. 1i). We and others have previously shown a similar activation of LMP2 and EBNA2 upon induction of lytic EBV by IgG cross-linking in Akata cells [27,28]. In striking contrast, none of the tested Zebularine concentrations exhibited an effect on latent EBV gene expression (Fig. 1j), suggesting that the failure of Zebularine to induce switching of latent to lytic EBV is not due to reinforcement of latent EBV gene expression. We therefore conclude that Zebularine has no effect on EBV gene expression in Akata cells, neither on lytic nor latent.

In the BL cell line Akata, both 5-Azacytidine and Zebularine are able to reactivate an important regulatory gene like E-cadherin, which when silenced by hypermethylation contributes to cell malignancy. Hypermethylation is also an important regulatory mechanism of EBV latency. This is emphasized by the fact that EBV can modulate the activity of DNA methyltransferases through the latent membrane protein LMP1, that can induce activation of DNA methyltransferases in epithelial carcinoma and lead to silencing of E-cadherin expression [29]. 5-Azacytidine and Zebularine act by different mechanisms [24]. Importantly, here we show that Zebularine, unlike 5-Azacytidine, does not disrupt EBV latency. Thus, Zebularine might be safer than 5-Azacytidine for the epigenetic treatment of cancers in EBV carriers and could also be employed to treat EBV-harboring tumors, since it does not induce switching from latent to lytic EBV a process linked to secondary EBV-associated malignancies.

Materials and methods
Cell lines
The human BL cell line Akata was cultured in RPMI 1640 medium (Invitrogen, Basel, Switzerland), supplemented with 10% heat-inactivated fetal calf serum, L-Glutamine (1%), penicillin (1 U/ml), streptomycin (1 µg/ml). The human bladder carcinoma cell line T24 was cultured in McCoy's medium supplemented with 10% fetal calf serum, L-Glutamine (1%), penicillin (1 U/ml), streptomycin (1 µg/ml). The cells were grown at 37°C in 5% CO_2 humidified atmosphere and split every third day. Akata cell line was a kind gift from Dr. A. Bell (Birmingham, UK), and T24 cell line was a kind gift from Dr. H. Wunderli-Allenspach (ETH Zürich, Switzerland). The optimal cell density (5×10^5 cells/ml) for experiments with Akata cells allowed logarithmic cell growth over the observation period.

DNA-methylase inhibitor treatments
5-Azacytidine was purchased from Sigma-Aldrich Chemie Gmbh (Buchs, Switzerland) as lyophilized powder and stored at -20°C. 5-Azacytidine solution was prepared fresh for each experiment in PBS at a concentration of 2.4 mg/ml (10 mM) and sterile filtered. Zebularine was purchased from Calbiochem (Merk Biosciences, Darmstadt, Germany) and stored at 4°C. Zebularine was dissolved in PBS at a concentration 28.5 mg/ml (120 mM), sterile fil-

tered and stored at 4°C. For each experiment with Akata cells, viable cells were counted by trypan-blue exclusion method and resuspended in fresh medium at 0.5 × 10^6 cells/ml. T24 cell line experiments were performed as described [18].

Quantitative real-time PCR analysis

RNA isolation was then performed by using Rneasy Mini Kit (Qiagen, Hombrechtikon, Switzerland) according to the manufacturer's protocol. Contaminating genomic DNA was removed by using DNA-free (Ambion Europe, Huntingdon, UK) according to the manufacturer's protocol. The RNA concentration was measured with an Eppendorf Bio Photometer (Vaudaux Eppendorf, Dübendorf, Switzerland). cDNA was prepared by reverse transcription of total RNA using the Omniscript RT-Kit (Quiagen) following the manufacturer's protocol. qRT-PCR was performed in a reaction volume of 10 µl with the ABI-TaqMan Master Mix with uracil-N-glycosylase (Applied Biosystems, Rotkreuz, Switzerland). Sequence information for the Taqman systems will be furnished upon request. mRNA expression of the target genes was normalized to the expression of the housekeeping gene HMBS [30]. The normalized transcription values correspond to $2^{-C_T(EBV)} \cdot C_T(HMBS) = 2^{-\Delta C_T}$, where C_T is the cycle threshold number that quantifies the target present.

Abbreviations

BL: Burkitt's lymphoma; EBV: Epstein-Barr virus; EBNA: EBV nuclear antigen; LMP: latent membrane protein; NPC: nasopharingeal carcinoma; qRT-PCR: quantitative real-time PCR; RT: retrotranscription.

Competing interests

The author(s) declare that they have no competing interests.

Authors' contributions

SPR carried out cell experiments and qRT-experiments and helped to draft the manuscript. MPR and MB carried out part of the cell experiments and qRT-experiments, participated in the experimental design and data analysis. CB designed and validated the qRT-PCR system for EBV. JAS carried out part of the cell experiments. DN and MB conceived the study, participated in its design and coordination, and drafted the manuscript. All authors read and approved the final manuscript.

Acknowledgements

Supported in part by the League against Cancer of the Kanton of Zurich

References

1. Esteller M: **DNA methylation and cancer therapy: new developments and expectations.** *Curr Opin Oncol* 2005, **17(1):**55-60.
2. Silverman LR, Demakos EP, Peterson BL, Kornblith AB, Holland JC, Odchimar-Reissig R, Stone RM, Nelson D, Powell BL, DeCastro CM, Ellerton J, Larson RA, Schiffer CA, Holland JF: **Randomized controlled trial of azacitidine in patients with the myelodysplastic syndrome: a study of the cancer and leukemia group B.** *J Clin Oncol* 2002, **20(10):**2429-2440.
3. Christman JK: **5-Azacytidine and 5-aza-2'-deoxycytidine as inhibitors of DNA methylation: mechanistic studies and their implications for cancer therapy.** *Oncogene* 2002, **21(35):**5483-5495.
4. Cihak A: **Biological effects of 5-azacytidine in eukaryotes.** *Oncology* 1974, **30(5):**405-422.
5. Notari RE, DeYoung JL: **Kinetics and mechanisms of degradation of the antileukemic agent 5-azacytidine in aqueous solutions.** *J Pharm Sci* 1975, **64(7):**1148-1157.
6. Kissinger LD, Stemm NL: **Determination of the antileukemia agents cytarabine and azacitidine and their respective degradation products by high-performance liquid chromatography.** *J Chromatogr* 1986, **353:**309-318.
7. Cohen JI: **Epstein-Barr virus infection.** *N Engl J Med* 2000, **343(7):**481-492.
8. Ben-Sasson SA, Klein G: **Activation of the Epstein-Barr virus genome by 5-aza-cytidine in latently infected human lymphoid lines.** *Int J Cancer* 1981, **28(2):**131-135.
9. Ernberg I, Falk K, Minarovits J, Busson P, Tursz T, Masucci MG, Klein G: **The role of methylation in the phenotype-dependent modulation of Epstein-Barr nuclear antigen 2 and latent membrane protein genes in cells latently infected with Epstein-Barr virus.** *J Gen Virol* 1989, **70:**2989-3002.
10. Masucci MG, Contreras-Salazar B, Ragnar E, Falk K, Minarovits J, Ernberg I, Klein G: **5-Azacytidine up regulates the expression of Epstein-Barr virus nuclear antigen 2 (EBNA-2) through EBNA-6 and latent membrane protein in the Burkitt's lymphoma line rael.** *J Virol* 1989, **63(7):**3135-3141.
11. Jansson A, Masucci M, Rymo L: **Methylation of discrete sites within the enhancer region regulates the activity of the Epstein-Barr virus BamHI W promoter in Burkitt lymphoma lines.** *J Virol* 1992, **66(1):**62-69.
12. Chan AT, Tao Q, Robertson KD, Flinn IW, Mann RB, Klencke B, Kwan WH, Leung TW, Johnson PJ, Ambinder RF: **Azacitidine induces demethylation of the Epstein-Barr virus genome in tumors.** *J Clin Oncol* 2004, **22(8):**1373-1381.
13. Feng WH, Cohen JI, Fischer S, Li L, Sneller M, Goldbach-Mansky R, Raab-Traub N, Delecluse HJ, Kenney SC: **Reactivation of latent Epstein-Barr virus by methotrexate: a potential contributor to methotrexate-associated lymphomas.** *J Natl Cancer Inst* 2004, **96(22):**1691-1702.
14. Hurd PJ, Whitmarsh AJ, Baldwin GS, Kelly SM, Waltho JP, Price NC, Connolly BA, Hornby DP: **Mechanism-based inhibition of C5-cytosine DNA methyltransferases by 2-H pyrimidinone.** *J Mol Biol* 1999, **286(2):**389-401.
15. Kim CH, Marquez VE, Mao DT, Haines DR, McCormack JJ: **Synthesis of pyrimidin-2-one nucleosides as acid-stable inhibitors of cytidine deaminase.** *J Med Chem* 1986, **29(8):**1374-1380.
16. Cheng JC, Matsen CB, Gonzales FA, Ye W, Greer S, Marquez VE, Jones PA, Selker EU: **Inhibition of DNA methylation and reactivation of silenced genes by zebularine.** *J Natl Cancer Inst* 2003, **95(5):**399-409.
17. Zhou L, Cheng X, Connolly BA, Dickman MJ, Hurd PJ, Hornby DP: **Zebularine: a novel DNA methylation inhibitor that forms a covalent complex with DNA methyltransferases.** *J Mol Biol* 2002, **321(4):**591-599.
18. Cheng JC, Yoo CB, Weisenberger DJ, Chuang J, Wozniak C, Liang G, Marquez VE, Greer S, Orntoft TF, Thykjaer T, Jones PA: **Preferential response of cancer cells to zebularine.** *Cancer Cell* 2004, **6(2):**151-158.
19. Lemaire M, Momparler LF, Bernstein ML, Marquez VE, Momparler RL: **Enhancement of antineoplastic action of 5-aza-2'-deoxycytidine by zebularine on L1210 leukemia.** *Anticancer Drugs* 2005, **16(3):**301-308.
20. Wiman KG, Magnusson KP, Ramqvist T, Klein G: **Mutant p53 detected in a majority of Burkitt lymphoma cell lines by monoclonal antibody PAb240.** *Oncogene* 1991, **6(9):**1633-1639.
21. Strathdee G: **Epigenetic versus genetic alterations in the inactivation of E-cadherin.** *Semin Cancer Biol* 2002, **12(5):**373-379.
22. Auerkari EI: **Methylation of tumor suppressor genes p16(INK4a), p27(Kip1) and E-cadherin in carcinogenesis.** *Oral Oncol* 2006, **42(1):**5-13.

23. Shaker S, Bernstein M, Momparler RL: **Antineoplastic action of 5-aza-2'-deoxycytidine (Dacogen) and depsipeptide on Raji lymphoma cells.** *Oncol Rep* 2004, **11(6):**1253-1256.
24. Stresemann C, Brueckner B, Musch T, Stopper H, Lyko F: **Functional diversity of DNA methyltransferase inhibitors in human cancer cell lines.** *Cancer Res* 2006, **66(5):**2794-2800.
25. Corn PG, Smith BD, Ruckdeschel ES, Douglas D, Baylin SB, Herman JG: **E-cadherin expression is silenced by 5' CpG island methylation in acute leukemia.** *Clin Cancer Res* 2000, **6(11):**4243-4248.
26. Packham G, Economou A, Rooney CM, Rowe DT, Farrell PJ: **Structure and function of the Epstein-Barr virus BZLF1 protein.** *J Virol* 1990, **64(5):**2110-2116.
27. Bernasconi M, Berger C, Sigrist JA, Bonanomi A, Sobek J, Niggli FK, Nadal D: **Quantitative profiling of housekeeping and Epstein-Barr virus gene transcription in Burkitt lymphoma cell lines using an oligonucleotide microarray.** *Virol J* 2006, **3:**43.
28. Yuan J, Cahir-McFarland E, Zhao B, Kieff E: **Virus and cell RNAs expressed during Epstein-Barr virus replication.** *J Virol* 2006, **80(5):**2548-2565.
29. Tsai CN, Tsai CL, Tse KP, Chang HY, Chang YS: **The Epstein-Barr virus oncogene product, latent membrane protein 1, induces the downregulation of E-cadherin gene expression via activation of DNA methyltransferases.** *Proc Natl Acad Sci U S A* 2002, **99(15):**10084-10089.
30. Bonanomi A, Kojic D, Giger B, Rickenbach Z, Jean-Richard-Dit-Bressel L, Berger C, Niggli FK, Nadal D: **Quantitative cytokine gene expression in human tonsils at excision and during histoculture assessed by standardized and calibrated real-time PCR and novel data processing.** *J Immunol Methods* 2003, **283(1-2):**27-43.

6.2 Silencing of latent membrane protein 2B (LMP2B) reduces susceptibility to activation of lytic Epstein-Barr virus in Burkitt's lymphoma Akata cells.

Rechsteiner MP, Berger C, Weber M, Sigrist JA, Nadal D, Bernasconi M.
Journal of General Virology, 88: 1454 – 1459 (2007).

Abstract

Epstein–Barr virus (EBV) latent membrane protein2A (LMP2A) blocks B-cell receptor (BCR) signalling after BCR cross-linking to inhibit activation of lytic EBV, and ectopically expressed LMP2B negatively regulates LMP2A. Here, it is demonstrated that silencing of LMP2B in EBV-harbouring Burkitt's lymphoma Akata cells results in reduced expression of EBV immediate – early lytic BZLF1 gene mRNA and late lytic gp350/220 protein upon BCR cross-linking. Similarly, reduction of lytic EBV activation was observed in Akata cells overexpressing LMP2A. In contrast, silencing of LMP2A expression resulted in higher lytic EBV mRNA and protein expression in BCR cross-linked Akata cells. These observations indicate a role for LMP2B distinct from that of LMP2A in regulation of lytic EBV activation in the host cell and support the hypothesis that LMP2B exhibits a negative-regulatory effect on the ability of LMP2A to maintain EBV latency by preventing the switch to lytic replication.

Short Communication

Silencing of latent membrane protein 2B reduces susceptibility to activation of lytic Epstein–Barr virus in Burkitt's lymphoma Akata cells

Markus P. Rechsteiner, Christoph Berger, Matthias Weber, Jürg A. Sigrist, David Nadal† and Michele Bernasconi†

Correspondence
David Nadal
david.nadal@kispi.unizh.ch

Michele Bernasconi
michele.bernasconi@
kispi.unizh.ch

Experimental Infectious Diseases and Cancer Research, University Children's Hospital of Zurich, Zurich, Switzerland

Epstein–Barr virus (EBV) latent membrane protein 2A (LMP2A) blocks B-cell receptor (BCR) signalling after BCR cross-linking to inhibit activation of lytic EBV, and ectopically expressed LMP2B negatively regulates LMP2A. Here, it is demonstrated that silencing of *LMP2B* in EBV-harbouring Burkitt's lymphoma Akata cells results in reduced expression of EBV immediate-early lytic *BZLF1* gene mRNA and late lytic gp350/220 protein upon BCR cross-linking. Similarly, reduction of lytic EBV activation was observed in Akata cells overexpressing LMP2A. In contrast, silencing of *LMP2A* expression resulted in higher lytic EBV mRNA and protein expression in BCR cross-linked Akata cells. These observations indicate a role for LMP2B distinct from that of LMP2A in regulation of lytic EBV activation in the host cell and support the hypothesis that LMP2B exhibits a negative-regulatory effect on the ability of LMP2A to maintain EBV latency by preventing the switch to lytic replication.

Received 12 December 2006
Accepted 4 January 2007

Epstein–Barr virus (EBV) is a human B-lymphotropic γ-herpesvirus that, following primary infection, persists latently in the host's memory B-cell pool for life and may switch periodically to lytic infection (Rickinson & Kieff, 2001). EBV is linked with malignancies including Burkitt's lymphoma (BL), Hodgkin's lymphoma, nasopharyngeal carcinoma and post-transplant lymphoproliferative diseases (Murray & Young, 2002), where it expresses different patterns of latency genes (Fruehling & Longnecker, 1997; Rowe, 1999). Latent EBV transforms B cells *in vitro* (Young & Murray, 2003). The two latent membrane proteins, LMP2A and LMP2B, are dispensable for this transformation (Longnecker et al., 1992; Speck et al., 1999), but seem to be involved in the maintenance of EBV latency.

Transcription of *LMP2A* and *LMP2B* is controlled by two promoters separated in the DNA by 3 kb (Sample et al., 1989). The two mRNAs encoding the proteins LMP2A and LMP2B have different 5′ exons followed by eight common exons. LMP2A contains an N-terminal cytoplasmic domain of 119 aa, with eight tyrosines that are phosphorylated in lymphoblastoid cell lines, 12 transmembrane domains and a C-terminal domain of 12 aa. LMP2B differs from LMP2A by the lack of the entire N-terminal cytoplasmic domain, which promotes B-cell survival by blocking B-cell receptor (BCR) signalling transduction through several signalling pathways (Fruehling et al., 1996; Fruehling & Longnecker,

1997; Longnecker et al., 1991; Miller et al., 1994b; Swart et al., 2000). Cross-linking of BCR on EBV-infected cells induces lytic EBV replication through transcriptional activation of the EBV immediate-early lytic gene *BZLF1*. In lymphoblastoid cell lines, LMP2A interferes with this process by blocking the activation of protein tyrosine kinases (Miller et al., 1994a, 1995). This mechanism is thought to prevent lytic EBV replication in latently infected B cells circulating in the body upon encounter of antigens or other ligands that may engage BCR (Portis et al., 2002). Indeed, LMP2A expression is found in EBV-infected tonsillar memory B cells *ex vivo* (Babcock & Thorley-Lawson, 2000; Babcock et al., 2000). Furthermore, B cells in *LMP2A*-transgenic mice show increased survival (Caldwell et al., 2000; Merchant et al., 2001). These observations suggest a central role for LMP2A to ensure persistence of EBV latency within the infected cell.

LMP2B, as for LMP2A, has been shown to promote spread and motility of epithelial cells (Allen et al., 2005), but little is known about the function of LMP2B in B cells. LMP2B co-localizes with LMP2A in the membrane, where the C termini of both splice variants can interact and regulate the activity of each other (Lynch et al., 2002; Matskova et al., 2001). Recently, LMP2B was shown to regulate LMP2A activity negatively when these genes were expressed in the EBV-negative BL cell line BJAB (Rovedo & Longnecker, 2007). Nevertheless, the role of LMP2B in the presence of EBV remains unknown.

†These authors contributed equally to this work.

We hypothesized that LMP2B exhibits a role distinct from that of LMP2A in activation of EBV lytic replication. To test our hypothesis, we compared the impact of *LMP2B* silencing with the impacts of LMP2A overexpression and *LMP2A* silencing on activation of EBV lytic replication in the EBV-harbouring BL cell line Akata upon BCR cross-linking (Takada, 1984). Akata cells retain an EBV gene expression pattern *in vitro* that closely resembles that found in BL biopsies, and are an established model for the study of activation of EBV lytic replication, which can be triggered effectively by BCR stimulation using cross-linking anti-IgG (Daibata *et al.*, 1990).

To silence expression of *LMP2B* specifically, we constructed a short hairpin (sh) RNA targeting exon 1 of *LMP2B*. The shRNA was designed by using the software RNAi Central (http://katahdin.cshl.org) and is available upon request. We cloned the shRNA into the lentiviral vector pSICOR (Ventura *et al.*, 2004), verified it by sequencing and named the construct pSICOR-LMP2B-68 (Table 1). After LMP2B-68 shRNA lentiviral production in HEK 293T cells (Graham *et al.*, 1977), we incubated wild-type Akata (Akata^{wt}) cells with concentrated virus-containing supernatant and amplified them for 1 month in culture using medium supplemented with G418 (0.4 mg ml^{-1}). To monitor uptake of pSICOR-LMP2B-68, we tested transduced Akata cells for expression of enhanced green fluorescence protein (EGFP) by flow cytometry. To obtain a homogeneous EGFP-expressing cell population (99 % purity), we enriched EGFP-expressing cells by fluorescence-activated cell sorting (FACS) twice and selected only for cells with high EGFP expression levels (Table 1). We independently transduced and selected three cell populations as described above to be used as biological replicates and designated them Akata-*LMP2B*^{shRNA}-pool 1, -pool 2 and -pool 3. We designed a control vector to encode a nonsense (scr) shRNA and generated Akata-*scr*^{shRNA} cells in the same way as Akata-*LMP2B*^{shRNA} cells.

To assess the efficiency and specificity of *LMP2B* silencing, we isolated total RNA from Akata-*LMP2B*^{shRNA} and control Akata-*scr*^{shRNA} cells. After cDNA synthesis, we used quantitative real-time (qRT)-PCR (Taqman) targeting an *LMP2B*-specific sequence (available upon request) to determine *LMP2B* mRNA expression levels. Results were normalized to housekeeping gene *hydroxymethylbilane synthase* (*HMBS*) mRNA expression, resulting in ΔC_t (cycle threshold) values. Akata cells are considered to be in latency I (EBNA1 expression only). However, even though no LMP2 protein can be detected, we observed low but significant levels of *LMP2A* and *LMP2B* mRNA expression (C_t range, 32–34; data not shown). Silencing of *LMP2B* in the three Akata-*LMP2B*^{shRNA} cell pools showed *LMP2B* mRNA expression levels to be 25.3 ± 2.3 % of those of Akata-*scr*^{shRNA} cells (Fig. 1a), but there was no change in *LMP2A* mRNA expression (not shown). The lack of available anti-LMP2B antibody precluded substantiation of the above qRT-PCR data by immunoblotting. Nevertheless, we considered the degree of silencing sufficient for our purposes, and the consistency of the degree of silencing justified the use of Akata-*LMP2B*^{shRNA}-pools 1, 2 and 3 as biological replicates in all subsequent experiments.

EBV lytic replication is initiated by upregulation of *BZLF1*. Thus, based on own previous observations (Bernasconi *et al.*, 2006), we determined *BZLF1* mRNA expression levels before and 6, 24, 48 and 72 h after BCR cross-linking by using qRT-PCR. ΔC_t values from unstimulated cells were subtracted from ΔC_t values from stimulated cells, resulting in $\Delta\Delta C_t$ values. mRNA expression of the vector control was set to 100 % and the percentages of reduction of mRNA expression in *LMP2B*-silenced cells were evaluated. *BZLF1* mRNA levels in *LMP2B*-silenced Akata-*LMP2B*^{shRNA} cells were 25–35 % of those in control Akata-*scr*^{shRNA} cells from 6 to 72 h after BCR cross-linking (Fig. 1b). Using flow cytometry, we found similar frequencies of surface IgG-positive cells in Akata-*LMP2B*^{shRNA} and Akata-*scr*^{shRNA}

Table 1. Characteristics of Akata cells used for silencing and overexpression experiments

wt, Wild type; shRNA, short hairpin RNA; ect, ectopic; EGFP, enhanced green fluorescent protein; sIgG, surface IgG; NM, not measured.

Experiment	Cell line	Vector construct	EGFP$^+$ (%)*	sIgG$^+$ (%)*	gp350/220 staining (% of cells)*		
					0 h	24 h	
						Stimulated	Unstimulated
Silencing	Akata^{wt}	None	NM	96			
Vector control	Akata *scr*^{shRNA}	pSICOR scrRNA	99	91	0.3 ± 0.1	1.7 ± 0.5	0.5 ± 0.2
LMP2B pool 1 3	Akata *LMP2B*^{shRNA}	pSICOR LMP2B 68	99 ± 1	90 ± 4	0.2 ± 0.2	0.3 ± 0.1	0.2 ± 0.1
LMP2A pool 1 3	Akata *LMP2A*^{shRNA}	pSICOR LMP2A	99 ± 1	84 ± 3	1.2 ± 0.6	2.2 ± 0.3	1.1 ± 0.5
Overexpression							
Vector control	Akata neo^{ect}	pEneo	NM	91			
LMP2A	Akata LMP2A^{ect}	pEneo LMP2A	NM	92			

*Values are presented as means ± SD.

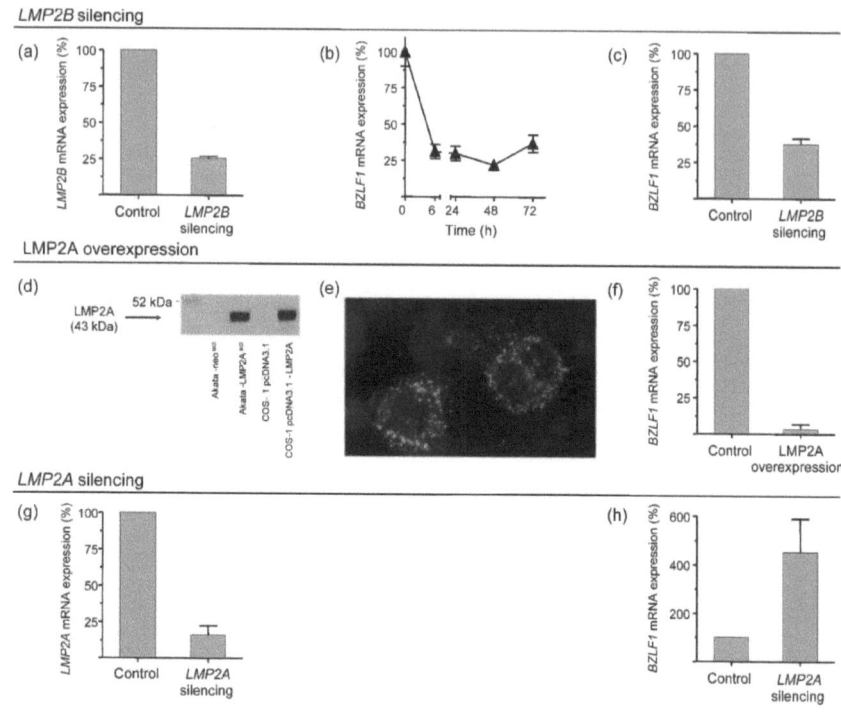

Fig. 1. *LMP2B* silencing, LMP2A overexpression and *LMP2A* silencing in Akata cells and impact on activation of EBV lytic replication upon BCR cross-linking. (a) Validation of *LMP2B* silencing: expression of *LMP2B* in Akata-*LMP2B*[shRNA] cells was measured by qRT-PCR. Data were normalized to those for *HMBS*, and expression of control Akata-*scr*[shRNA] cells was set to 100 % (means and SD of pools). (b) Impact of *LMP2B* silencing on activation of EBV lytic replication upon BCR cross-linking. Cells (0.5×10^6) were seeded and treated with or without polyclonal rabbit anti-human IgG (0.1 μg μl^{-1}) for 3 h. After stimulation, cells were centrifuged and suspended in fresh medium. Immediate-early lytic *BZLF1* mRNA levels were measured at the indicated times before and after BCR cross-linking with a specific Taqman system. The mRNA expression of control Akata cells was set to 100 % for each time point, and the percentage reduction of mRNA expression in *LMP2B*-silenced Akata cells was evaluated. One representative experiment of three carried out in triplicate is shown. (c) *LMP2B* silencing in Akata cells resulted in decreased activation of lytic EBV 24 h after BCR cross-linking. Data shown represent the means and SD of three independent experiments. (d, e) Validation of LMP2A overexpression by (d) immunoblotting and (e) immunostaining. Immunoreactive proteins were detected by the specific rat anti-LMP2A antibody 8C3. (f) Expression of EBV immediate-early lytic *BZLF1* mRNA in Akata-LMP2A[ect] cells showed a decrease 24 h after BCR cross-linking compared with control. Means and SD of three independent stimulations are shown. (g) Validation of *LMP2A* silencing by qRT-PCR in Akata-*LMP2B*[shRNA] cells (mean and SD of pools) and Akata-*scr*[shRNA] cells. (h) *LMP2A* silencing in Akata-*LMP2A*[shRNA] cells resulted in increased activation of EBV lytic replication 24 h after BCR cross-linking. Data shown represent the means and SD of three independent experiments.

cells (Table 1). This excluded the possibility that the differences in *BZLF1* mRNA expression levels upon BCR cross-linking were due to differences in surface IgG expression. Thus, the reduced *BZLF1* mRNA expression in Akata-*LMP2B*[shRNA] cells was probably a direct consequence of *LMP2B* silencing.

To substantiate the above qRT-PCR results, we stained Akata-*LMP2B*[shRNA] and Akata-*scr*[shRNA] cells before and 24 h after BCR cross-linking with a fluorescein isothiocyanate-labelled antibody against EBV late lytic gp350/220 protein in three independent experiments performed in triplicate (Table 1). Both unstimulated Akata-*LMP2B*[shRNA] and

Akata-scr^{shRNA} cells showed a similar low basal percentage of cells staining for gp350/220 (mean±SD, 0.3±0.1%). Consistent with the qRT-PCR data, 24 h after BCR cross-linking, Akata-$LMP2B^{shRNA}$ cells showed a 4- to 5-fold lower number of cells positive for gp350/220 than Akata-scr^{shRNA} cells (0.3±0.1% versus 1.7±0.5%). Thus, upon BCR cross-linking, induction of EBV lytic replication in $LMP2B$-silenced Akata-$LMP2B^{shRNA}$ cells is lower than in Akata-scr^{shRNA} cells, not only at the mRNA expression level of the immediate-early lytic gene $BZLF1$, but also at the level of the late lytic protein gp350/220, indicating a reduced susceptibility of $LMP2B$-silenced EBV-harbouring cells to activation of EBV lytic replication.

Next, we reasoned that if LMP2B regulates LMP2A negatively, which prevents activation of lytic EBV, overexpression of LMP2A should yield outcomes similar to those of $LMP2B$ silencing. Therefore, we amplified the sequence encoding LMP2A from the vector pSG5-LMP2 (Sample et al., 1989) by PCR and cloned the PCR product via PmeI/XhoI into the Moloney murine leukemia virus-derived pEneo bicistronic expression vector containing an internal ribosome entry site with a neomycin selection marker (Schaefer et al., 2001). Positive clones were verified by sequencing. The parental pEneo plasmid was used as control vector. Akata^{wt} cells were transfected by electroporation with the pEneo-LMP2A expression vector or the parental vector pEneo. After 2 days recovery, the transfected cells were subjected to G418 selection. Stably transfected cells emerged after 2–3 weeks. Expression of $LMP2A$ mRNA was confirmed by qRT-PCR (not shown) and immunoblotting showing expression of the correct-sized protein at 43 kDa (Fig. 1c). These cells were named Akata-LMP2A^{ect}, and the control cells Akata-neo^{ect} (Table 1). Immunofluorescence staining showed expression of LMP2A in all Akata-LMP2A^{ect} cells, with heterogeneous high and low LMP2A expression levels reflecting a polyclonal population (Fig. 1d), but no expression in the control Akata-neo^{ect} cells (not shown). These populations showed no up- or down-regulation of $LMP2B$ mRNA expression by qRT-PCR (not shown) and similar levels of surface IgG (Table 1), confirming that LMP2A overexpression had not affected $LMP2B$ mRNA or surface IgG expression.

To compare susceptibility to activation of lytic EBV in LMP2A-overexpressing Akata cells with the above-assessed activation in $LMP2B$-silenced Akata cells, we stimulated Akata-LMP2A^{ect} and control Akata-neo^{ect} cells by BCR cross-linking. We chose 24 h after BCR cross-linking for the comparison because $LMP2B$-silenced Akata and control cells had shown a suitable difference in $BZLF1$ mRNA expression at 24 h (Fig. 1b, c). Stimulated and unstimulated Akata cells were collected and examined by qRT-PCR for $BZLF1$ mRNA expression. The data were normalized to $HMBS$ mRNA and further normalized to mRNA levels in unstimulated cells as mentioned above. The results are presented as ratios of stimulated over unstimulated Akata cells. As expected from published data (Fukuda & Longnecker, 2005; Konishi et al., 2001), $BZLF1$ mRNA

expression in LMP2A-overexpressing cells was reduced to 3.3±5.7% of that in control cells in three independent experiments (Fig. 1f). This superior reduction, compared with the reduction to 33.3±6.7% seen in $LMP2B$-silenced cell pools (Fig. 1c), was probably intrinsic to the nature of the experiments, with overexpression of LMP2A being more effective than LMP2B silencing. Nevertheless, the reduced $BZLF1$ mRNA expression upon BCR cross-linking in EBV-harbouring $LMP2B$-silenced and LMP2A-overexpressing cells indicated that LMP2B modulates LMP2A negatively in preventing activation of EBV lytic replication.

To verify our results by using an opposite approach, we constructed a silencing pSICOR vector specific for $LMP2A$, targeting exon 1 of $LMP2A$ (Stewart et al., 2004), and transduced it virally into Akata^{wt} cells as described above for $LMP2B$ silencing to obtain pools 1, 2 and 3 of Akata-$LMP2A^{shRNA}$ cells (Table 1). Akata-$LMP2A^{shRNA}$ cell pools showed $LMP2A$ mRNA expression levels of 15.9±11.1% of those in control cells (Fig. 1g), but no effect on $LMP2B$ mRNA expression levels (not shown), confirming the specificity of silencing. To assess the effect of $LMP2A$ silencing on induction of EBV lytic replication, we measured $BZLF1$ mRNA expression levels 24 h following BCR cross-linking in the three biological replicates and compared the levels with those in the corresponding control cells. Activation of EBV lytic replication in $LMP2A$-silenced cells was 2- to 6-fold higher than in control cells, as illustrated by the increase of $BZLF1$ mRNA to 552.3±89.9% compared with vector-control Akata-scr^{shRNA} cells (Fig. 1h). Increased activation of EBV lytic replication in $LMP2A$-silenced cells was confirmed at the protein level by the measurement of the expression of gp350/220 in Akata-$LMP2A^{shRNA}$ cells (Table 1). Akata-$LMP2A^{shRNA}$ cells expressed higher basal levels of gp350/220 before stimulation (1.2±0.6%) and at 24 h unstimulated (1.1±0.5%) than did Akata-scr^{shRNA} cells (0.3±0.1 and 0.4±0.2%, respectively). Twenty-four hours after stimulation, the detected envelope protein reached levels of up to 2.2±0.3% in Akata-$LMP2A^{shRNA}$-pool 1 cells, compared with 1.7±0.5% of Akata-scr^{shRNA} cells. Thus, stimulated Akata-$LMP2A^{shRNA}$ cells show a 1.3-fold increase of gp350/220 expression compared with Akata-scr^{shRNA} cells, similar to the data obtained from qRT-PCR. This indicates that silencing of $LMP2A$ increases the susceptibility to activation of EBV lytic replication. Therefore, silencing of $LMP2B$ and $LMP2A$ exhibits opposite effects on susceptibility to activation of EBV lytic replication.

LMP2A plays a relevant role in controlling the switch from EBV latency to lytic replication in B cells through modulation of the activity of cellular kinases, including the Src family of phosphotyrosine kinases (Mancao et al., 2005; Portis et al., 2004), and calcium mobilization following BCR cross-linking. This results in a decreased activation of lytic EBV. LMP2B lacks an N-terminal signalling domain and cannot therefore influence any signalling cascade directly. Rovedo & Longnecker (2007) showed that LMP2B and LMP2A can interact with each other in the EBV-negative BL cell line

BJAB, resulting in decreased phosphorylation of the LMP2A cytoplasmic N-terminal domain and the block of cytoplasmic calcium release upon BCR cross-linking.

Here, we show that silencing of *LMP2B* reduces activation of EBV lytic replication in the BL cell line Akata, as does overexpression of LMP2A. This indicates that LMP2B decreases the block of LMP2A on BCR activation. In contrast, specific silencing of *LMP2A* in Akata cells had exactly the opposite effect of increasing induction of lytic EBV replication upon stimulation, as documented by *BZLF1* mRNA expression and gp350/220 protein expression. Hence, given that LMP2A prevents lytic EBV activation (Miller et al., 1994b, 1995), our results support the notion that LMP2B negatively affects LMP2A regulation of activation of lytic EBV upon BCR cross-linking.

Akata cells are known to maintain latency I in culture (Takada, 1984) and express low levels of LMP2A (Konishi et al., 2001), and are negative for LMP2B protein expression when probed by immunoblotting. More sensitive tools like Southern–PCR (Tao et al., 1998) or qRT-PCR, as shown here, are able to detect low mRNA expression levels of both *LMP2A* and *LMP2B* in exponentially growing Akata cells. We were able to detect LMP2A after immunoprecipitation of resting Akata^{wt} cells, but could not observe any quantitative changes upon activation of lytic EBV (M. Bernasconi & J. A. Sigrist, unpublished observation). Low levels of LMP2A do not seem sufficient to block activation upon BCR cross-linking in Akata cells (Konishi et al., 2001). However, our results indicate that, for as low as the protein expression level is, both LMP2A and LMP2B influence the susceptibility to activation of lytic EBV infection.

In conclusion, our results suggest that LMP2B adds a novel layer of complexity to the regulation of lytic EBV infection in B cells. Together with the observations made in the EBV-negative cell line BJAB (Rovedo & Longnecker, 2007), we suggest that LMP2B under some circumstances impacts on the activity of LMP2A, resulting in increased susceptibility to activation of lytic EBV replication through modulation of BCR and downstream signalling.

Acknowledgements

We thank Brigitte Kappeler and Ursina Cagienard for vector construction and virus production, Nicole Köchli for establishment of qRT PCR assays and Dr C. Esslinger for help in flow cytometry and FACS. We also thank Professor T. Jacks for kindly providing the pSICOR plasmids, Dr A. Bell for providing Akata cells and Professor R. Longnecker for the LMP2A plasmid. The study was supported by the League against Cancer of the Canton of Zurich and by UBS AG by order of a client.

References

Allen, M. D., Young, L. S. & Dawson, C. W. (2005). The Epstein Barr virus encoded LMP2A and LMP2B proteins promote epithelial cell spreading and motility. *J Virol* **79**, 1789 1802.

Babcock, G. J. & Thorley-Lawson, D. A. (2000). Tonsillar memory B cells, latently infected with Epstein Barr virus, express the restricted pattern of latent genes previously found only in Epstein Barr virus associated tumors. *Proc Natl Acad Sci U S A* **97**, 12250 12255.

Babcock, G. J., Hochberg, D. & Thorley-Lawson, A. D. (2000). The expression pattern of Epstein Barr virus latent genes in vivo is dependent upon the differentiation stage of the infected B cell. *Immunity* **13**, 497 506.

Bernasconi, M., Berger, C., Sigrist, J. A., Bonanomi, A., Sobek, J., Niggli, F. K. & Nadal, D. (2006). Quantitative profiling of house keeping and Epstein Barr virus gene transcription in Burkitt lymphoma cell lines using an oligonucleotide microarray. *Virol J* **3**, 43.

Caldwell, R. G., Brown, R. C. & Longnecker, R. (2000). Epstein Barr virus LMP2A induced B cell survival in two unique classes of EmuLMP2A transgenic mice. *J Virol* **74**, 1101 1113.

Daibata, M., Humphreys, R. E., Takada, K. & Sairenji, T. (1990). Activation of latent EBV via anti IgG triggered, second messenger pathways in the Burkitt's lymphoma cell line Akata. *J Immunol* **144**, 4788 4793.

Fruehling, S. & Longnecker, R. (1997). The immunoreceptor tyrosine based activation motif of Epstein Barr virus LMP2A is essential for blocking BCR mediated signal transduction. *Virology* **235**, 241 251.

Fruehling, S., Lee, S. K., Herrold, R., Frech, B., Laux, G., Kremmer, E., Grasser, F. A. & Longnecker, R. (1996). Identification of latent membrane protein 2A (LMP2A) domains essential for the LMP2A dominant negative effect on B lymphocyte surface immunoglobulin signal transduction. *J Virol* **70**, 6216 6226.

Fukuda, M. & Longnecker, R. (2005). Epstein Barr virus (EBV) latent membrane protein 2A regulates B cell receptor induced apoptosis and EBV reactivation through tyrosine phosphorylation. *J Virol* **79**, 8655 8660.

Graham, F. L., Smiley, J., Russell, W. C. & Nairn, R. (1977). Character istics of a human cell line transformed by DNA from human adenovirus type 5. *J Gen Virol* **36**, 59 74.

Konishi, K., Maruo, S., Kato, H. & Takada, K. (2001). Role of Epstein Barr virus encoded latent membrane protein 2A on virus induced immortalization and virus activation. *J Gen Virol* **82**, 1451 1456.

Longnecker, R., Druker, B., Roberts, T. M. & Kieff, E. (1991). An Epstein Barr virus protein associated with cell growth transformation interacts with a tyrosine kinase. *J Virol* **65**, 3681 3692.

Longnecker, R., Miller, C. L., Miao, X. Q., Marchini, A. & Kieff, E. (1992). The only domain which distinguishes Epstein Barr virus latent membrane protein 2A (LMP2A) from LMP2B is dispensable for lymphocyte infection and growth transformation in vitro; LMP2A is therefore nonessential. *J Virol* **66**, 6461 6469.

Lynch, D. T., Zimmerman, J. S. & Rowe, D. T. (2002). Epstein Barr virus latent membrane protein 2B (LMP2B) co localizes with LMP2A in perinuclear regions in transiently transfected cells. *J Gen Virol* **83**, 1025 1035.

Mancao, C., Altmann, M., Jungnickel, B. & Hammerschmidt, W. (2005). Rescue of 'crippled' germinal center B cells from apoptosis by Epstein Barr virus. *Blood* **106**, 4339 4344.

Matskova, L., Ernberg, I., Pawson, T. & Winberg, G. (2001). C terminal domain of the Epstein Barr virus LMP2A membrane protein contains a clustering signal. *J Virol* **75**, 10941 10949.

Merchant, M., Caldwell, R. G. & Longnecker, R. (2000). The LMP2A ITAM is essential for providing B cells with development and survival signals in vivo. *J Virol* **74**, 9115 9124.

Miller, C. L., Lee, J. H., Kieff, E., Burkhardt, A. L., Bolen, J. B. & Longnecker, R. (1994a). Epstein Barr virus protein LMP2A regulates reactivation from latency by negatively regulating tyrosine kinases involved in sIg mediated signal transduction. *Infect Agents Dis* 3, 128 136.

Miller, C. L., Lee, J. H., Kieff, E. & Longnecker, R. (1994b). An integral membrane protein (LMP2) blocks reactivation of Epstein Barr virus from latency following surface immunoglobulin crosslinking. *Proc Natl Acad Sci U S A* 91, 772 776.

Miller, C. L., Burkhardt, A. L., Lee, J. H., Stealey, B., Longnecker, R., Bolen, J. B. & Kieff, E. (1995). Integral membrane protein 2 of Epstein Barr virus regulates reactivation from latency through dominant negative effects on protein tyrosine kinases. *Immunity* 2, 155 166.

Murray, P. G. & Young, L. S. (2002). The role of the Epstein Barr virus in human disease. *Front Biosci* 7, d519 d540.

Portis, T., Cooper, L., Dennis, P. & Longnecker, R. (2002). The LMP2A signalosome a therapeutic target for Epstein Barr virus latency and associated disease. *Front Biosci* 7, d414 d426.

Portis, T., Ikeda, M. & Longnecker, R. (2004). Epstein Barr virus LMP2A: regulating cellular ubiquitination processes for maintenance of viral latency? *Trends Immunol* 25, 422 426.

Rickinson, A. B. & Kieff, E. (2001). Epstein Barr Virus. In *Fields Virology*, 4th edn, pp. 2575 2627. Edited by D. M. Knipe & P. M. Howley. Philadelphia, PA: Lippincott Williams & Wilkins.

Rovedo, M. & Longnecker, R. (2007). Epstein Barr virus latent membrane protein 2B (LMP2B) modulates LMP2A activity. *J Virol* 81, 84 94.

Rowe, D. T. (1999). Epstein Barr virus immortalization and latency. *Front Biosci* 4, D346 D371.

Sample, J., Liebowitz, D. & Kieff, E. (1989). Two related Epstein Barr virus membrane proteins are encoded by separate genes. *J Virol* 63, 933 937.

Schaefer, B. C., Mitchell, T. C., Kappler, J. W. & Marrack, P. (2001). A novel family of retroviral vectors for the rapid production of complex stable cell lines. *Anal Biochem* 297, 86 93.

Speck, P., Kline, K. A., Cheresh, P. & Longnecker, R. (1999). Epstein Barr virus lacking latent membrane protein 2 immortalizes B cells with efficiency indistinguishable from that of wild type virus. *J Gen Virol* 80, 2193 2203.

Stewart, S., Dawson, C. W., Takada, K., Curnow, J., Moody, C. A., Sixbey, J. W. & Young, L. S. (2004). Epstein Barr virus encoded LMP2A regulates viral and cellular gene expression by modulation of the NF kappaB transcription factor pathway. *Proc Natl Acad Sci U S A* 101, 15730 15735.

Swart, R., Ruf, I. K., Sample, J. & Longnecker, R. (2000). Latent membrane protein 2A mediated effects on the phosphatidylinositol 3 kinase/Akt pathway. *J Virol* 74, 10838 10845.

Takada, K. (1984). Cross linking of cell surface immunoglobulins induces Epstein Barr virus in Burkitt lymphoma lines. *Int J Cancer* 33, 27 32.

Tao, Q., Robertson, K. D., Manns, A., Hildesheim, A. & Ambinder, R. F. (1998). Epstein Barr virus (EBV) in endemic Burkitt's lymphoma: molecular analysis of primary tumor tissue. *Blood* 91, 1373 1381.

Ventura, A., Meissner, A., Dillon, C. P., McManus, M., Sharp, P. A., Van Parijs, L., Jaenisch, R. & Jacks, T. (2004). Cre lox regulated conditional RNA interference from transgenes. *Proc Natl Acad Sci U S A* 101, 10380 10385.

Young, L. S. & Murray, P. G. (2003). Epstein Barr virus and oncogenesis: from latent genes to tumours. *Oncogene* 22, 5108 5121.

6.3 Latent membrane protein 2B regulates susceptibility to activation of lytic Epstein-Barr virus infection.

Rechsteiner MP, Berger C, Zauner L,. Sigrist JA, Weber M, Longnecker R, Bernasconi M, Nadal D. Journal of Virology, 82: 1739-1747 (2008).

Abstract

The B-lymphotropic Epstein-Barr virus (EBV) encodes two isoforms of the latent membrane protein 2 (LMP2), LMP2A and LMP2B, which are expressed during latency in B-cells. The function of LMP2B is largely unknown, whereas LMP2A blocks B-cell receptor (BCR) signaling transduction and induction of lytic EBV infection, thereby promoting B-cell survival. Transfection experiments of LMP2B in EBV-negative B-cells and the silencing of LMP2B in EBV-harboring Burkitt's lymphoma-derived Akata cells suggest that LMP2B interferes with the function of LMP2A, but the role of LMP2B in the presence of functional EBV has not been established. Here, LMP2B, LMP2A, or both were overexpressed in EBV-harboring Akata cells to study the function of LMP2B. Overexpression of LMP2B increased the magnitude of EBV switching from its latent to its lytic form upon BCR cross-linking, as indicated by a more enhanced upregulation and expression of EBV lytic genes and significantly increased production of transforming EBV compared to Akata vector control cells or LMP2A overexpressing cells. Moreover, LMP2B lowered the degree of BCR cross-linking required to induce lytic EBV infection. Finally, LMP2B co-localized with LMP2A as demonstrated by immunoprecipitation and immunofluorescence and restored calcium mobilization upon BCR cross-linking, a signaling process inhibited by LMP2A. Thus, our findings suggest that LMP2B negatively regulates the function of LMP2A in preventing the switch from latent to lytic EBV replication.

Latent Membrane Protein 2B Regulates Susceptibility to Induction of Lytic Epstein-Barr Virus Infection[▽]

Markus P. Rechsteiner,[1] Christoph Berger,[1] Ludwig Zauner,[1] Jürg A. Sigrist,[1] Matthias Weber,[1] Richard Longnecker,[2] Michele Bernasconi,[1]† and David Nadal[1]*†

Experimental Infectious Diseases and Cancer Research, Division of Infectious Diseases and Hospital Epidemiology, University Children's Hospital of Zurich, CH-8032 Zurich, Switzerland,[1] and Department of Microbiology and Immunology, Feinberg School of Medicine, Northwestern University, Chicago, Illinois 60611[2]

Received 8 August 2007/Accepted 24 November 2007

The B-lymphotropic Epstein-Barr virus (EBV) encodes two isoforms of latent membrane protein 2 (LMP2), LMP2A and LMP2B, which are expressed during latency in B cells. The function of LMP2B is largely unknown, whereas LMP2A blocks B-cell receptor (BCR) signaling transduction and induction of lytic EBV infection, thereby promoting B-cell survival. Transfection experiments on LMP2B in EBV-negative B cells and the silencing of LMP2B in EBV-harboring Burkitt's lymphoma-derived Akata cells suggest that LMP2B interferes with the function of LMP2A, but the role of LMP2B in the presence of functional EBV has not been established. Here, LMP2B, LMP2A, or both were overexpressed in EBV-harboring Akata cells to study the function of LMP2B. The overexpression of LMP2B increased the magnitude of EBV switching from its latent to its lytic form upon BCR cross-linking, as indicated by a more-enhanced upregulation and expression of EBV lytic genes and significantly increased production of transforming EBV compared to Akata vector control cells or LMP2A-overexpressing cells. Moreover, LMP2B lowered the degree of BCR cross-linking required to induce lytic EBV infection. Finally, LMP2B colocalized with LMP2A as demonstrated by immunoprecipitation and immunofluorescence and restored calcium mobilization upon BCR cross-linking, a signaling process inhibited by LMP2A. Thus, our findings suggest that LMP2B negatively regulates the function of LMP2A in preventing the switch from latent to lytic EBV replication.

Epstein-Barr virus (EBV) is a ubiquitous B-lymphotropic gammaherpesvirus which persists after primary infection latently in the host for life and may switch periodically to its lytic form (28). In vitro, EBV undergoes very efficient growth transformation and immortalizes infected B cells by latent infection, resulting in lymphoblastoid cell lines (LCLs) expressing a limited number of viral genes, including six viral nuclear antigens (EBNAs) and latent membrane protein 1 (LMP1) and LMP2 (30). The ability to transform B cells implicates EBV as the culprit for a variety of malignancies, including Burkitt's lymphoma, Hodgkin's disease, and posttransplant lymphoproliferative disease (8, 24, 38). In vivo, EBV persists in latently infected memory B cells circulating in the peripheral blood (30). These latently infected cells do not express EBNAs or LMP1, but may express LMP2 (1, 2). Since LMP2 has no transformation capacity (12), this may suggest a pivotal role of LMP2 in the regulation of the balance between latent and lytic EBV.

Transcription of *LMP2* is controlled by two promoters separated in the viral DNA by 3 kb (31). Two mRNAs that have different 5′ exons followed by eight common exons encode two distinct proteins, LMP2A and LMP2B, respectively. LMP2A contains an N-terminal cytoplasmic domain of 119 amino acids with eight tyrosines that are phosphorylated in LCLs, 12 transmembrane domains, and a C-terminal domain of 12 amino acids. LMP2A blocks B-cell receptor (BCR) signal transduction through specific phosphotyrosine motifs in its N-terminal domain and promotes B-cell survival. This function is dependent on the expression level of LMP2A (1, 2, 5, 6, 15, 21, 35). LMP2B lacks the entire N-terminal cytoplasmic domain. A recent work using transfection of LMP2B to EBV-negative cells has suggested possible roles for LMP2B. LMP2B colocalized with LMP2A in the membrane where the C terminus of both splice variants can interact and regulate the activity of each other (17). Furthermore, LMP2B was shown to negatively regulate LMP2A activity by interfering with its aggregation (29). Another study revealed protein domains of LMP2B which are required for intra- and extracellular localization and self-aggregation (37), which raised the question of whether the function of LMP2B in EBV is bound to its localization independently of LMP2A. Nevertheless, whether and how LMP2B is involved in the regulation of latent and lytic EBV infection in B cells harboring the functional virus remains a largely unresolved question.

Burkitt's lymphoma-derived Akata cells provide an optimal model to study the balance between latent and lytic EBV. Specifically, lytic EBV infection can be initiated in Akata cells by cross-linking their BCR using anti-immunoglobulin G (anti-IgG) (36). Importantly, upon induction of lytic EBV infection, the majority of viral genes are expressed (3, 39). Since these EBV genes could have an impact on the function of LMP2B, we used Akata cells to investigate the function of LMP2B in cells harboring functional EBV. Recently, we found that the

* Corresponding author. Mailing address: Experimental Infectious Diseases and Cancer Research, Division of Infectious Diseases and Hospital Epidemiology, University Children's Hospital of Zurich, Zurich, Switzerland. Phone: 41-44-266-7250. Fax: 41-44-266-7082. E-mail: david.nadal@kispi.uzh.ch.
† Contributed equally.
▽ Published ahead of print on 5 December 2007.

silencing of *LMP2B* reduces susceptibility to induction of lytic EBV infection upon BCR cross-linking (27). This result indicated a role of LMP2B distinct from that of LMP2A in the regulation of EBV lytic activation. In this work, we further pursue the hypothesis that LMP2B exhibits a negative-regulatory effect on LMP2A maintenance of EBV latency. Thus, we compared the effects of overexpression of LMP2B and LMP2A on the susceptibility to induction of lytic EBV infection and on cellular signaling pathways in Akata cells.

MATERIALS AND METHODS

Cell lines and primary cells. The Burkitt's lymphoma cell line Akata (36) was grown in RPMI 1640 supplemented with 10% fetal calf serum, L-glutamine (2 mM), penicillin (100 U/ml), and streptomycin (100 μg/ml). Akata cells were a kind gift of A. Bell (Birmingham, United Kingdom). Akata cells transfected with the plasmids pEneo (33), pEneo-LMP2A (27), and pEneo-FLAG-LMP2B, named Akata-vector (27), Akata-LMP2A (27), and Akata-LMP2B pools 1 to 3, respectively, were cultured in the same medium supplemented with 0.4 mg/ml G418 (Promega, Mannheim, Germany). Akata-cre cells that stably overexpress the regulatable creER^{T2} recombinase (9) integrated into the vector pcDNA3.1 were cultured in the same medium supplemented with 0.4 mg/ml G418 (Promega, Mannheim, Germany). Cord blood mononuclear cells (CBMC) were obtained from heparinized blood by Ficoll-Hypaque gradient centrifugation (Amersham Biosciences Europe GmbH, Otelfingen, Switzerland) and washed with phosphate-buffered saline (Gibco, Invitrogen Life Sciences, Basel, Switzerland). Informed consent was obtained from parturient women. The Zurich institutional ethics committee approved the collection and use of clinical material. B95.8 cells were cultured in Dulbecco's minimal essential medium supplemented with 10% fetal calf serum, L-glutamine (2 mM), penicillin (100 U/ml), and streptomycin (100 μg/ml) (23).

Plasmids. The sequence coding for LMP2B was PCR amplified from the vector pSG5-LMP2 (15, 31) with following primers, including cloning adapters and 3× FLAG for LMP2B tagging: FLAG-LMP2B-F (5′-CGCGTTTAAACAT GGACTACAAAGACCATGACGGTGATTATAAAGATCATGATATCGAT TACAAGGATGACGATGACAAGAATCCAGTATGCCTGCCTG-3′) and LMP2-Rev (5′-GCGCTCGAGTTATACAGTGTTGCGATATGGGGTC-3′). The PCR product was cloned via PmeI/XhoI into the Moloney murine leukemia virus-derived pEneo bicistronic expression vector containing an internal ribosome entry site with a neomycin selection marker (33), resulting in the vectors pEneo-FLAG-LMP2B and pEneo-LMP2A (27). Positive clones were verified by sequencing. The parental pEneo plasmid was used as the control vector.

Transfection. Cells (1×10^6) were electroporated with 2 μg of the pEneo, pEneo-LMP2A, or pEneo-FLAG-LMP2B plasmid with Nucleofector II (Amaxa GmbH, Cologne, Germany) with Buffer T and the program A-23. Electroporated cells were allowed to recover for 2 days and were then selected with 0.8 mg/ml G418 (Promega) for 2 to 3 weeks until resistant cells arose. These cells were named Akata-vector, Akata-LMP2A, and Akata-LMP2B pools 1 to 3, respectively. One month after selection, cells were supplemented with 0.4 mg/ml G418 and used for experiments. To generate double-transfected Akata cells, either stable Akata-LMP2B cells were electroporated transiently ($_t$) with the vector pEneo-LMP2A (named 2B + A$_t$) or Akata-LMP2A cells were electroporated transiently with the vector pEneo-FLAG-LMP2B (named 2A + B$_t$).

Immunoblot analysis. Total cellular protein extracts were prepared by disruption of cells in radioimmunoprecipitation assay lysis buffer (150 mM NaCl, 1% NP-40, 0.5% deoxycholate, 0.1% sodium dodecyl sulfate [SDS], and 50 mM Tris, pH 7.5). After denaturation for 10 min in 4× loading LDS buffer (Invitrogen, Basel, Switzerland), samples were separated on a 10% Bis-Tris gel (Invitrogen) and transferred to a nitrocellulose membrane (Schweizer & Schell Bioscience GmbH, Dassel, Germany). Membranes were blocked with 5% low-fat milk in 1× phosphate-buffered saline (PBS)–0.1% Tween 20 and incubated with either mouse anti-FLAG M2 (Sigma, St. Louis, MO), rat anti-LMP2A (clone 14B7) (5), or anti-c-*myc* (A-14; Santa Cruz Biotech, Inc., Santa Cruz, CA) antibody overnight at 4°C. Immunoreactive proteins were detected by the secondary antibodies against mouse and rabbit, respectively (Cell Signaling Technology, Danvers, MA) and an enhanced chemiluminescence detection kit (SuperSignal West Femto; Perbio Science Switzerland S.A., Lausanne, Switzerland).

IP. Total cellular protein extracts were prepared by disruption of 5×10^6 cells in Tris nondenaturing lysis buffer (150 mM NaCl, 1% Triton X-100, 1 mM EDTA, and 50 mM Tris, pH 7.5), 2 mM NaF, and 2 mM Orthovanadate (all from Sigma). Isolated proteins were immunoprecipitated with a Sigma immunoprecipitation (IP) kit according to the manufacturer's instructions. IPs were performed with the same antibodies used for immunoblotting or without an antibody.

Immunostaining. Cells (5×10^4) were centrifuged by Cytospin on double Cytofunnel glass slides (Thermo, Waltham, MA) and fixed with methanol for 10 min at −20°C. Cells were permeabilized with 1% Triton X-100 in 1× PBS for 20 min at room temperature. Immunoreactive proteins were detected with a rat anti-LMP2A antibody, 14B7 (1:100), and a secondary Alexa 488-labeled goat anti-rat IgG antibody diluted 1:200 (Molecular Probes, Invitrogen). FLAG-tagged LMP2B was detected with anti-FLAG M2 from Sigma (1:500) and a secondary Alexa 594-labeled goat anti-mouse IgG antibody diluted 1:200 (Molecular Probes, Invitrogen). BZLF1 was detected with anti-BZLF1 (Argene, North Massapequa, NY) diluted 1:100 and probed with the same secondary antibody used for FLAG detection.

Flow cytometry. To evaluate the surface IgG (sIgG) content of transfected cells for later stimulation experiments with BCR cross-linking, cells were fixed in 4% paraformaldehyde (Sigma) and stained with a phycoerythrin-labeled anti-human IgG1,κ antibody (BD Biosciences, Basel, Switzerland). A phycoerythrin-labeled anti-mouse IgG1,κ antibody (BD Biosciences) was used as an isotype control. To determine the percentage of cells in which EBV was activated by BCR cross-linking, 0.5×10^6 cross-linked and non-cross-linked cells were stained with a fluorescein isothiocyanate (FITC)-labeled antiviral gp350/220 antibody diluted 1:10 (Biodesign International, Saco, ME) and analyzed by flow cytometry (FC-500; Beckmann-Coulter, Krefeld, Germany).

BCR cross-linking of Akata cells. Akata cells were split to 0.5×10^6 cells/ml 24 h before BCR cross-linking. Cells (0.5×10^6/ml) were then BCR cross-linked with 0.1 μg/μl polyclonal rabbit anti-human-IgG (Dako, Zug, Switzerland) for 3 h and suspended afterwards in fresh RPMI 1640. Cross-linked and non-cross-linked cells were collected for subsequent analyses.

qRT-PCR. Total RNA was extracted from 0.5×10^6 cells with an RNeasy kit from Qiagen (Hombrechtikon, Switzerland). DNase [DNA-free; Ambion (Europe), Huntington, Cambridgeshire, United Kingdom] treatment was performed before cDNA synthesis with an Omniscript RT kit (Qiagen). Quantitative real-time PCR (qRT-PCR) was done with validated TaqMan systems for the housekeeping gene *HMBS* and the lytic EBV genes *BZLF1*, *BXLF1*, and *LMP2* (14) on an ABI 7200 (Applied Biosystems). TaqMan data were analyzed using SDS 2.2 (Applied Biosystems), and mRNA expression was normalized to *HMBS* mRNA, resulting in threshold cycle (ΔC_T) values. ΔC_T values were further normalized by dividing "cross-linked" by "not cross-linked" values, resulting in $\Delta\Delta C_T$ values. qRT-PCR data for control vector $\Delta\Delta C_T$ were set to 100% and LMP2B- or LMP2A-overexpressing cells were compared to it.

Transformation assay. Fifty thousand freshly isolated CBMC per well were seeded in a 96-well plate. Culture supernatants were filtered through a 0.45-μm polyvinylidene difluoride Millex-HV filter (Millipore Corporation, MA). Fifty microliters of filtered culture supernatant of cells 24 h after anti-IgG cross-linking or no cross-linking was added to a final volume of 100 μl per well. A total of 10 wells for each filtered culture supernatant was plated and inoculated. Filtered supernatant from B95.8 served as the positive control, whereas the negative control was CBMC cultured with medium only (23). The transformation capacity was monitored by counting the wells after 6 weeks, when growth and clustering of cells could be observed (34). The percentage of transformation was calculated by setting 10 transformed wells to 100% and by normalization to the transformation capacity of the supernatant of cells that were not cross-linked, representing the spontaneous activation of EBV in Akata cells. Statistics were done with Prism 4 (GraphPad Software, Inc.).

Calcium mobilization. Cells (5×10^6) were stained with Fluo-3 (6 μM final concentration) and Fura-Red (15 μM final concentration; both from Invitrogen) for 45 min in RPMI 1640 at 37°C. After a washing step with 1× PBS, cells were stored at room temperature in the dark. Before measurement, cells were incubated for 5 min at 37°C. Calcium mobilization was measured by adding ionomycin (2 μg/ml final concentration; Invitrogen) as the control and anti-IgG at the same concentration as in stimulation experiments (100 μg/ml) by using a FC-500 (Beckmann-Coulter) with an argon laser at 488 nm. Fluorescent emission was recorded at 520 nm (Fluo-3) and 670 nm (Fura-Red), and the Fluo-3/Fura-Red ratio was plotted against time. The baseline was recorded prior to anti-IgG addition for 30 s and for 5 min after BCR cross-linking. The increase over the baseline level was calculated for the time of peak of calcium mobilization (t_p) by using FlowJo 5.7.2 software. The percentage of responding cells was calculated for the time slice from t_p to $t_{p\ +\ 2\ min}$. As an additional control, Akata-cre cells were stimulated and the calcium mobilization was measured.

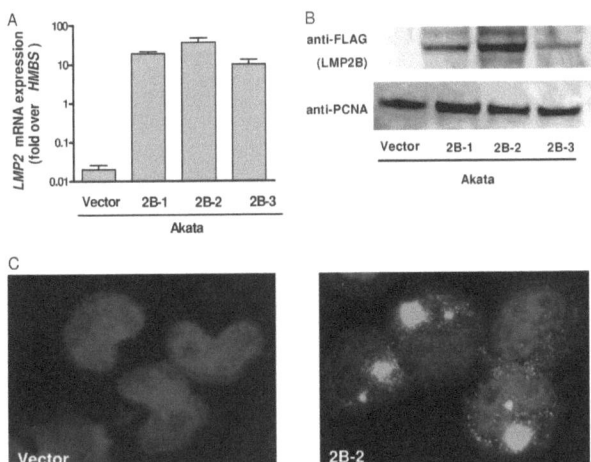

FIG. 1. Generation of LMP2B-overexpressing Akata cells. (A) Overexpression of LMP2B pools 1 to 3 (2B-1, 2B-2, 2B-3) by qRT-PCR using specific TaqMan systems targeting *HMBS* and *LMP2* mRNA, respectively. (B) Immunoblot of FLAG-LMP2B pools 1 to 3 (2B-1, 2B-2, 2B-3). (C) Immunostaining of FLAG-LMP2B in Akata-vector control cells and Akata-LMP2B pool 2 (2B-2).

RESULTS

Construction of LMP2B-overexpressing Akata cells. In order to investigate the effects of LMP2B on LMP2A and the switch from latent to lytic EBV replication, we first constructed EBV-harboring Akata cells overexpressing either LMP2B or LMP2A (27) and Akata cells with the vector control (27). Given that no specific antibody against LMP2B exists, we chose to tag LMP2B with a 3× FLAG sequence at the N terminus. The tag was placed at the N terminus, since it has been suggested that clustering of LMP2A and LMP2B occurs over the common C termini and that LMP2B influences the activity of its LMP2A isoform only when they colocalize (18, 29). As the transfection efficiency of B cells is low with common protocols, we decided to establish Akata cell pools stably overexpressing LMP2B, LMP2A, or a control vector. Thus, Akata cells were transfected independently with pEneo-FLAG-LMP2B, pEneo-LMP2A, or the control vector pEneo alone, as described in Materials and Methods. After neomycin selection, stable overexpression of LMP2B was verified for all three independently transfected Akata cell pools at the RNA level by qRT-PCR and at the protein level by immunoblotting and immunostaining. The three LMP2B-overexpressing cell pools (Akata-LMP2B pools 1, 2, and 3) showed different levels of overexpression of LMP2B after transfection (Fig. 1A). The mRNA expression levels correlated with protein levels, whereby Akata-LMP2B pool 1 showed a medium level, pool 2 a high level, and pool 3 the lowest level of LMP2B mRNA and protein, respectively (Fig. 1B). Immunostaining was done with Akata-LMP2B pool 2. Most overexpressed LMP2B localized to cytosolic compartments, whereas smaller amounts were detected in the plasma membrane (Fig. 1C). Furthermore, all cell lines were stained for sIgG and were found to express sIgG in similar percentages (Table 1). Thus, similar prerequisites for susceptibility to stimulation by BCR cross-linking with anti-IgG were ensured in the distinct cell lines.

LMP2B overexpression increases the magnitude of EBV lytic activation after BCR cross-linking. To assess the distinct effects of LMP2B and LMP2A on lytic activation of EBV in

TABLE 1. Characteristics of Akata cells used[a]

Cell line	Vector construct	% sIgG+ cells	% Cells activated by gp350/220 staining		
			0 h	24 h	
				Cross-linked	Not cross-linked
Akata[b]	None	96 ± 1	ND	ND	ND
Akata-vector[b]	pEneo	92 ± 2	0.30 ± 0.11	4.62 ± 0.06	0.58 ± 0.09
Akata-LMP2B[c]	pEneo-FLAG-LMP2B	88 ± 4	0.36 ± 0.20	5.42 ± 0.94	0.69 ± 0.23
Akata-LMP2A[b]	pEneo-LMP2A	92 ± 1	0.24 ± 0.05	1.00 ± 0.81	0.34 ± 0.13

[a] ND, not detected.
[b] Values are presented as means ± SD from three independent experiments.
[c] Values are presented as means ± SD from pools 1 to 3.

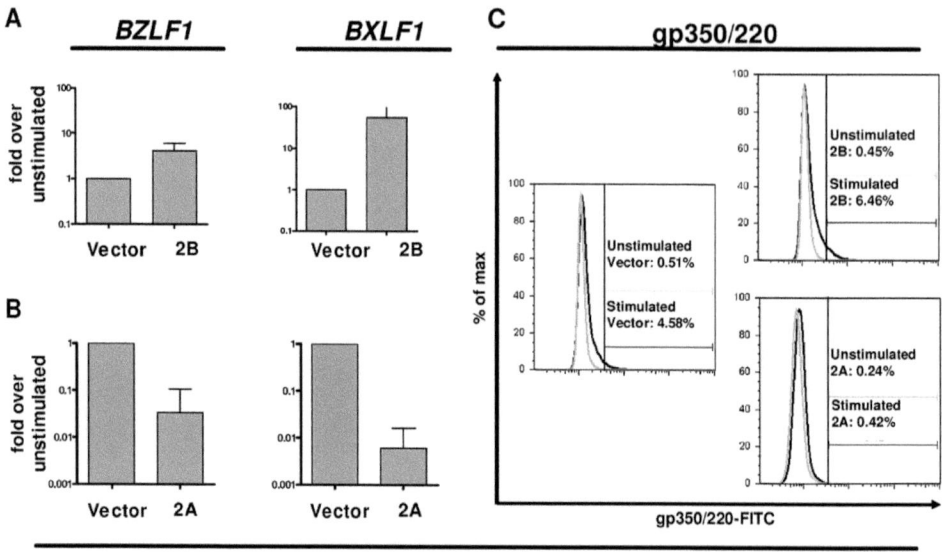

FIG. 2. LMP2B overexpression increases the magnitude of EBV lytic activation after BCR cross-linking, whereas LMP2A overexpression results decreased magnitude. qRT-PCR with specific systems for *HMBS*, *BZLF1*, and *BXLF1* mRNA, respectively, for Akata-vector control, Akata-LMP2B (A), and Akata-LMP2A (B) 24 h after BCR cross-linking. Means and standard deviations (SD) of qRT-PCR results are from three independent stimulation experiments on one representative polyclonal population. (C) Flow cytometry for gp350/220-FITC-labeled unstimulated (gray line) or stimulated (black line) cells 24 h after BCR cross-linking. One representative measurement is shown for Akata-vector control, Akata-LMP2B, and Akata-LMP2A cells with gp350/220-FITC-positive cells gated and indicated as percentages. Means and SD for three independent experiments are summarized in Table 1.

Akata cells, we stimulated Akata-LMP2B cells or Akata-LMP2A cells and the corresponding Akata-vector control cells by BCR cross-linking. After 24 h, cross-linked and non-cross-linked cells were collected and examined by qRT-PCR for expression of the immediate-early lytic gene *BZLF1* and the early lytic gene *BXLF1* encoding the viral thymidine kinase. The data were normalized to *HMBS* mRNA expression and are presented as ratios of cross-linked to non-cross-linked cells (Fig. 2). Akata-LMP2B cells showed mRNA expression levels of *BZLF1* and *BXLF1* that increased 4-fold and 55-fold, respectively (Fig. 2A). By contrast and as expected, transcription levels of lytic EBV genes were reduced in Akata-LMP2A cells, where expression of *BZLF1* and *BXLF1* mRNAs was reduced by 97% and 99%, respectively (Fig. 2B). To confirm these results at the protein level, we stained cells before and 24 h after BCR cross-linking with a FITC-labeled antiviral gp350/220 antibody in three independent stimulations. Indeed, as determined by flow cytometry, Akata-LMP2B cell pools expressed up to 5.4-fold- and 4.6-fold-higher gp350/220 levels than Akata-LMP2A cells and Akata-vector control cells, respectively (Fig. 2C; Table 1).

LMP2B-overexpressing Akata cells produce more infectious EBV than control cells upon BCR cross-linking. To verify the complete activation of the EBV lytic cycle following BCR cross-linking, the production of infectious EBV was monitored by the transformation of primary human B cells (34). Following BCR cross-linking of Akata-LMP2B, Akata-LMP2A, and Akata-vector control cells, supernatants were prepared from three independent experiments and added to freshly isolated CBMC to determine the transformation capacity of the infectious EBV produced. After normalization to non-cross-linked cells, the transformation capacities of supernatants from Akata-vector control cells were 67%, but those from Akata-LMP2B-cell pools were up to 100% ($P = 0.0356$), in contrast to the 0% transformation capacity of supernatants from Akata-LMP2A cells ($P = 0.0089$; Fig. 3).

Overexpression of LMP2B decreases the degree of BCR stimulation required to induce lytic EBV infection, in contrast to overexpression of LMP2A. LMP2A blocks BCR signaling, thereby impeding EBV lytic activation (6). It is not clear how the expression level of LMP2A influences the degree of BCR cross-linking (BCR activation) required to induce lytic EBV infection and how this is affected by LMP2B overexpression. Therefore, we assessed the magnitude of EBV lytic activation as a function of the anti-IgG dose to engage BCR by cross-linking Akata-vector, Akata-LMP2B, or Akata-LMP2A cells with increasing concentrations of anti-IgG. To quantify the activation of EBV lytic infection, mRNA expression of *BZLF1*

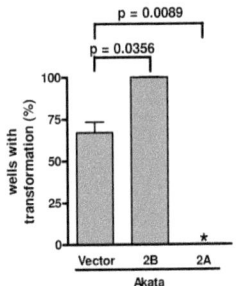

FIG. 3. More infectious EBV is produced in LMP2B-overexpressing Akata cells than in the control. Isolated CBMC were infected with supernatant from Akata-vector control, Akata-LMP2A, or Akata-LMP2B pools 1 to 3 collected 24 h after stimulation by BCR cross-linking. The transformation capacity was monitored by counting the wells after 6 weeks, at which time growth and clustering of cells indicated transformation. The percentage of transformation was calculated by setting 10 wells showing signs of transformation to 100% and by normalization to the transformation capacity of the supernatant of the corresponding BCR non-cross-linked control cells, representing the spontaneous EBV lytic activation in Akata cells. Means and SD are from three independent stimulation experiments with subsequent collection of supernatant and infection of CBMC. t tests were performed with a 95% confidence interval. *, no wells showed signs of transformation.

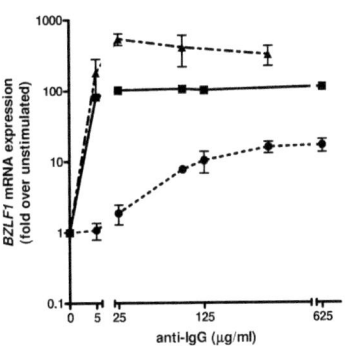

FIG. 4. Overexpression of LMP2B decreases the degree of BCR stimulation required to induce lytic EBV infection, in contrast to overexpression of LMP2A. BZLF1 mRNA expression in Akata-vector control (■), Akata-LMP2A (●), or Akata-LMP2B (▲) 24 h after BCR cross-linking using increasing doses of anti-IgG. Means and SD are from three independent stimulation experiments on one representative polyclonal population.

at 24 h after BCR cross-linking was measured (Fig. 4). Cross-linked Akata-vector control cells compared to non-cross-linked control cells showed an almost 100-fold increase of BZLF1 mRNA expression with the lowest anti-IgG concentration of 5 μg/ml and around 100-fold-higher peak BZLF1 mRNA expression levels with anti-IgG concentrations of 25 μg/ml or higher. Akata-LMP2B cells showed a similar but greater increase in BZLF1 mRNA expression and around five-fold-higher peak levels than Akata-vector cells with anti-IgG concentrations of 25 μg/ml or higher. By contrast, Akata-LMP2A cells required anti-IgG concentrations of at least 25 μg/ml to show an increase in BZLF1 mRNA expression and an anti-IgG concentration of 625 μg/ml to show maximal BZLF1 mRNA expression levels, which were around 10-fold lower than peak expression levels in Akata-vector cells. Thus, cells with higher expression levels of LMP2A required higher doses of anti-IgG to induce an EBV lytic activation, which was still of a considerably lower magnitude than that for Akata-vector control cells. These results suggest that the expression level of LMP2A has an impact on the amount of BCR cross-linking required to induce lytic EBV infection and that higher expression levels of LMP2A can be overridden, though only partially, with a higher degree of BCR cross-linking. On the other hand, higher LMP2B expression levels seemed to lower the degree of BCR cross-linking required to induce EBV lytic activation and to increase the magnitude of inducible EBV lytic activation.

LMP2B physically interacts with LMP2A before and after BCR cross-linking in Akata cells. To investigate whether overexpressed LMP2B physically interacts with endogenous LMP2A, we isolated whole-cell protein extracts from Akata-LMP2B pool 2 (2B-2) and Akata-vector control cells with a subsequent pull-down IP of LMP2A. Subsequently, we performed immunoblotting against FLAG tags and LMP2A (Fig. 5A). Indeed, coimmunoprecipitated LMP2B was detected by anti-FLAG in Akata-LMP2B cells but not in Akata-vector control cells, whereas endogenous LMP2A was detected in both. Control IPs, with an anti-c-myc antibody or without antibody and subsequent immunoblotting against c-myc or FLAG (Fig. 5B and C) showed no unspecific pull-down, confirming the specificity of the IPs, despite the overexpression of FLAG-LMP2B.

Next, to elucidate in which compartment LMP2B and LMP2A localize, we transfected Akata-LMP2A (2A) transiently with FLAG-LMP2B (B_t) (indicated as 2A + B_t) and immunostained LMP2A or FLAG-LMP2B for fluorescent microscopy. The images shown in Fig. 6B suggest partial colocalization of both LMP2 isoforms in the same cellular compartments (Fig. 6B). Additionally, we found an accumulation of LMP2B in the cytosolic region, as seen in stable Akata-LMP2B and described above (Fig. 1C). To determine if there is a relocalization of LMP2A or LMP2B upon BCR cross-linking, we double-stained Akata-LMP2A cells transiently transfected with FLAG-LMP2B (2A + B_t) for FLAG-LMP2B and for LMP2A (Fig. 6C), and for BZLF1 and LMP2A (Fig. 6D) after BCR cross-linking. An immunofluorescence analysis indicated a rather modest shift of LMP2A and LMP2B into the cytosol after BCR cross-linking, but still-adequate amounts of both LMP2s were located in the same compartments as before BCR cross-linking.

LMP2B restores calcium mobilization in LMP2A-overexpressing Akata cells. It has been previously established that LMP2A blocks calcium mobilization induced by BCR cross-linking (20–22). To investigate the impact of LMP2B overexpression on calcium mobilization, we determined the calcium levels before (baseline) and after BCR cross-linking, monitoring the kinetics for 5 min in Akata-vector control, Akata-LMP2B pool 2 (2B-2), and Akata-LMP2A (2A) cells, respectively. Additionally, Akata-cre cells overexpressing creER^{T2}

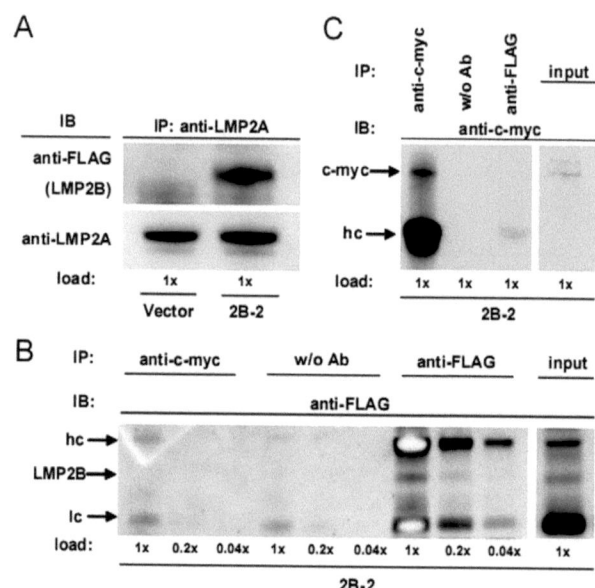

FIG. 5. LMP2B coimmunoprecipitates with LMP2A. Whole-cell protein lysates of Akata-LMP2B pool 2 (2B-2) and the Akata-vector control were immunoprecipitated (IP) with anti-LMP2A (A). The IPs were separated on a SDS gel and immunoblotted (IB) against FLAG and LMP2A. The heavy band in the LMP2A immunoblot represents the heavy Ig chain of the mouse antibody used for pull-down, whereas the lower, narrow band represents the equal amount of LMP2A pulled down in 2B-2 and vector input lysates. (B) The input lysate of 2B-2 was split into IPs without antibody, against c-myc, and FLAG and immunoblotted (three dilutions; 1×, 0.2×, 0.04×) against FLAG. No unspecific pull-down with anti-c-myc was observed due to the overexpression of FLAG-LMP2B. (C) The same IPs as those used in panel B were loaded on a SDS gel and immunoblotted against c-myc to verify that the IP was working. The upper band (65 kDa) and the lower band (63 kDa) in the input lysate of 2B-2 represent two forms of c-myc.

recombinase in the cytosol were stimulated and monitored in parallel to exclude any epiphenomena due merely to overexpression which could influence calcium mobilization. Calcium mobilization reached up to 3-fold, 3.3-fold, and 3.5-fold peaks compared to baseline levels after BCR cross-linking in Akata-vector control cells, Akata-cre cells, and Akata-LMP2B cells, respectively (Fig. 7). Next, we generated double transfectants by electroporation of Akata-LMP2B cells transiently with the vector pEneo-LMP2A (2B + A$_t$) as described in Materials and Methods and measured the calcium mobilization after BCR cross-linking. We observed not only a decrease of calcium mobilization from 3.5-fold to 1.9-fold in Akata-LMP2B cells but also a decrease of responding cells from 90% to 74%. These results are in agreement with previous studies (20–22). The calcium mobilization in Akata-LMP2A cells revealed the same low calcium mobilization and percentage of responding cells as observed in the double-transfected 2B + A$_t$ cells (1.8-fold and 77%, respectively). To address the question of whether it is possible to rescue the phenotype of Akata-vector control cells, we transiently transfected Akata-LMP2A cells with the vector pEneo-FLAG-LMP2B (2A + B$_t$). Interestingly, the calcium mobilization was restored to Akata-vector control cell levels from 1.8- to 2.9-fold after BCR cross-linking.

Additionally, responding cells increased from 77% to 82% in double-transfected 2A + B$_t$ cells (Fig. 7).

DISCUSSION

In this work, we investigated the impact of LMP2B on the potential of LMP2A to maintain EBV in its latent state. We demonstrate that LMP2B increases the magnitude of EBV switching from its latent to its lytic form upon BCR cross-linking, lowers the degree of BCR cross-linking required to provoke this switching, and is involved in augmenting signaling via calcium mobilization upon BCR cross-linking in Akata cells harboring functional EBV. These observations suggest a negative regulatory effect of LMP2B on the ability of LMP2A to block BCR signaling, thereby preventing EBV from switching from latent to lytic infection in B cells.

Although LMP2A and LMP2B are similar in their structure, the lack of the signaling amino-terminal domain in LMP2B indicates distinct functions for these two proteins. Indeed, the overexpression of LMP2B in Akata cells resulted in higher mRNA expression of immediate-early and early lytic EBV genes upon BCR cross-linking, whereas the overexpression of LMP2A results in lower mRNA expression in these genes.

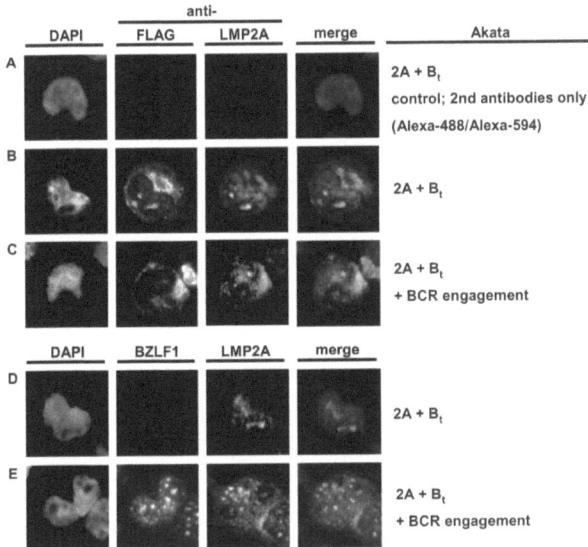

FIG. 6. Overexpressed LMP2B and LMP2A colocalize before and after BCR cross-linking. (A) Negative control for secondary antibodies. (B) To investigate where LMP2B and LMP2A localize, we transiently transfected Akata-LMP2A cells with FLAG-LMP2B (2A + B$_t$) and stained for LMP2A and FLAG-LMP2B. To determine if there occurs a relocalization of LMP2A or LMP2B upon BCR cross-linking, we stained the double-transfected Akata cells (2A + B$_t$) for FLAG-LMP2B and for LMP2A (C) and for BZLF1 and LMP2A (D) 3 h after BCR cross-linking (E). DAPI, 4',6'-diamidino-2-phenylindole.

Moreover, LMP2B overexpression leads as well to production of more EBV envelope protein gp350/220 and functional virus than do LMP2A-overexpressing or control Akata cells upon BCR cross-linking. These findings are compatible with our previous observation that silencing of *LMP2B* in Akata cells reduces the susceptibility of these cells to undergo EBV lytic activation induced by BCR cross-linking (27). Thus, our current and previous data provide evidence that LMP2B is involved in the regulation of EBV switching from latent to lytic infection EBV in B cells harboring the whole virus in its latent form.

The overexpression of LMP2B did not result in spontaneous switching of latent to lytic EBV. Nevertheless, the higher magnitude of EBV lytic activation in LMP2B-overexpressing Akata cells than that in control Akata cells upon BCR cross-linking with similar doses of anti-IgG suggested that LMP2B exerts its mode of action through lowering the required degree of BCR cross-linking and thus BCR signaling needed. Since LMP2A blocks BCR signaling (5, 6, 12, 15, 21, 29, 30, 35), we addressed the fundamental question of whether the magnitude of EBV lytic activation at given expression levels of the LMP2s depends on the dose of anti-IgG required to cross-link BCR, i.e., the degree of BCR cross-linking. Indeed, although increasing doses of anti-IgG elevated the levels of activation of lytic EBV in LMP2A-overexpressing Akata cells until they reached a plateau, peak levels of induced lytic EBV in these cells were around at least 10-fold lower than in control Akata cells or around 30- to 50-fold lower than in LMP2B-overexpressing Akata cells. This result suggests that both endogenous and overexpressed LMP2A is able to reduce BCR signaling very effectively and cannot be completely counteracted, even by saturated levels of anti-IgG added for cross-linking. Thus, the amount of overexpressed LMP2B was able to decrease the activity of endogenous LMP2A on BCR signaling but could not abolish it completely in whole-EBV-containing cells.

An important question to be addressed was if there is an interaction of LMP2A and LMP2B in Akata cells harboring EBV and, if so, where the two isoforms of LMP2 colocalize. The physical interaction between LMP2A and LMP2B was verified by pulling down FLAG-LMP2B with endogenous LMP2A. Our immunostaining results suggest an accumulation of LMP2B in intracellular compartments and to a lesser extent on the plasma membranes of Akata cells harboring whole EBV. Lynch et al. (17) reported that transiently expressed LMP2B localized to perinuclear regions and colocalized with transiently or constitutively expressed LMP2A in EBV-negative BJAB cells or LCL B95-8CR, respectively. Studies using HEK 293 cells overexpressing full-length or deletion mutants of LMP2A revealed a clustering signal of LMP2A at the C terminus leading to homodimerization (18). As LMP2A and LMP2B share eight exons and the C terminus, Rovedo and Longnecker (29) hypothesized that LMP2B colocalizes with LMP2A, forming heterodimers, and subsequently negatively regulates LMP2A activity, leading to decreased degradation of

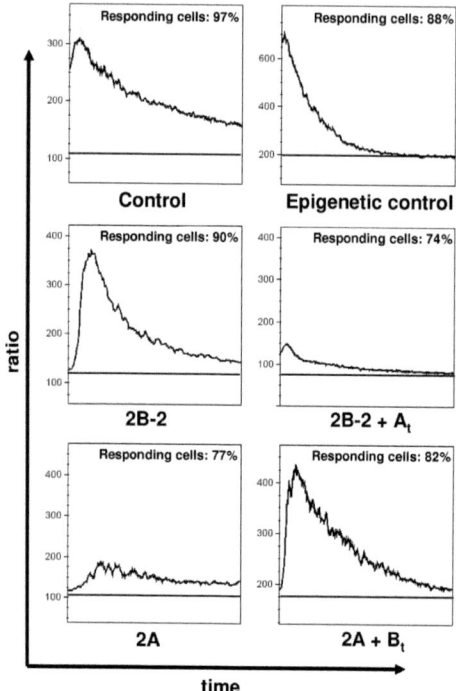

FIG. 7. LMP2B restores calcium mobilization in LMP2A-overexpressing Akata cells. Calcium levels were determined before and after BCR cross-linking, and the kinetics were measured for 5 min. Upper panels, calcium mobilization after BCR cross-linking in Akata control cells and, as an additional control, in Akata cells with epigenetic overexpression of an unspecific protein in the cytosol (see Materials and Methods). Middle panels, calcium mobilization after BCR cross-linking in Akata-LMP2B cells without (2B) and with (2B + A_t) transiently transfected LMP2A. Lower panels, calcium mobilization after BCR cross-linking in Akata-LMP2A cells without (2A) and with (2A + B_t) transiently transfected FLAG-LMP2B. Baselines were measured just before BCR cross-linking. The percentage of responding cells was calculated as described in Materials and Methods.

the tyrosine kinase Lyn. A more-recent study showed that when tagged LMP2B was overexpressed in BJAB cells or HEK 293T cells, LMP2B was found exclusively in intracellular perinuclear compartments (29, 37), a result which is in apparent contrast with the results of the aforementioned study. When LMP2B was truncated at any domain, it resulted in localization to the cell surface. Based on these results taken together, one can hypothesize that the major impact of LMP2B on LMP2A takes place in endosomes, where it interferes either with the activity of LMP2A and subsequent ubiquitination and degradation of Lyn or with the trafficking of LMP2A back to the plasma membrane.

An immunofluorescence analysis of LMP2A and LMP2B suggested a colocalization of LMP2A and LMP2B in Akata cells overexpressing both proteins. We detected a rather modest shift of LMP2B and LMP2A into the cytosol, which suggests their internalization after BCR cross-linking. Nevertheless, a large amount of both LMP2s remains detectable on the plasma membrane, demonstrating an intact turnover process. Moreover, this experiment allowed us to exclude the possibility of misfolded and degraded protein in the endoplasmic reticulum due to overexpression, as has been reported in earlier studies (10, 19). It is known that LMP2A aggregates in lipid rafts, assembling as a signalosome which enables a transient interaction with the tyrosine kinases Syk and Lyn with a subsequent block of the BCR signal (5–7, 15, 16, 21, 25, 26, 35). One can hypothesize that after BCR cross-linking, the anti-IgG/BCR complex is internalized together with closely located lipid rafts and LMP2A signalosomes. If there is an additional function of LMP2A in preventing the whole complex from being transported again to the cell membrane, in this way blocking continuous stimulation, one can hypothesize that there is a loss of LMP2A at the cell surface and an accumulation in endosomes located in the cytosol after BCR cross-linking. LMP2B, which is found in cytosolic compartments, may intervene in this step, disrupting homodimerized LMP2A and restoring the turnover.

As demonstrated here for the first time, calcium mobilization upon BCR cross-linking is dependent on the expression level of LMP2B in EBV-harboring Akata cells. As expected from previous reports (20–22), we observed virtually no calcium mobilization in LMP2A-overexpressing cells upon BCR cross-linking. By contrast, after transient transfection of LMP2B into LMP2A-overexpressing Akata cells, calcium mobilization after BCR cross-linking is increased to levels comparable to those observed for Akata cells overexpressing LMP2B. Conversely, we measured a reduced calcium mobilization in LMP2B-overexpressing Akata cells transiently transfected with LMP2A. As transiently transfected vectors expressing the gene of interest lead to high levels of protein, the dominant effect on the stably transfected Akata cells was predictable. Three different signaling pathways which are activated upon BCR cross-linking in Akata cells have been analyzed: (i) calcium mobilization through phosphatidylinositol 3-kinase, (ii) c-Jun N-terminal kinase activation through Syk and Lyn signaling, and (iii) ERK1/2 phosphorylation through the RAS protein (4). Nevertheless, whether LMP2B is involved partially or throughout all these signaling cascades, taking a key regulatory function upstream, remains unknown. Rovedo and Longnecker showed recently that in the EBV-negative B-cell line BJAB, ectopically expressed LMP2B decreases the activity of LMP2A by alteration of the phosphorylation status (29). Thus, LMP2B would function at an initial step of BCR signaling to restore BCR signal transduction which was blocked by LMP2A. As a more downstream read-out, they chose to measure the calcium mobilization in BJAB cells upon BCR cross-linking. As has previously been shown, the overexpression of LMP2A nearly abolished calcium mobilization (20–22). According to the hypothesis of BCR signal restoration by LMP2B, ectopic overexpression of both splice variants of LMP2 together resulted in the phenotype of BJAB transfected with vector control only.

LMP2B may have important functions not only in the modulation of latent and lytic EBV infection in tumor cells or memory B cells in the periphery. As was reported previously, LMP2A is expressed in newly infected naïve B cells before latency is established and serves as a tonic signal for survival. This scenario might be true for B cells with crippled or a total loss of BCR expression, leading in the worst case to Hodgkin's lymphoma (11, 13). In contrast, if a naïve B cell which has a functional BCR is newly infected and receives the survival signal, the additional signal of LMP2A might resemble in total an activated BCR, forcing EBV to lytic infection. In the presence of LMP2B, the signal of LMP2A would be downregulated, not leading to activated lytic EBV as was suggested previously for high levels of LMP2A (32).

In conclusion, the data presented here provide evidence that LMP2B is involved in the regulation of switching from latent to lytic EBV in B cells harboring functional EBV. Based on our present and previous findings for Akata cells (27) together with observations made for the EBV-negative cell line BJAB (29), we suggest that LMP2B has an impact on the activity of LMP2A, resulting in increased susceptibility to induction of lytic EBV infection through modulation of BCR and downstream signaling.

ACKNOWLEDGMENTS

This work was supported by the Cancer League of the Canton of Zurich, the Edoardo, R. Giuseppe and Christina Sassella Foundation, and the Novartis Foundation for Research in Medical Biology.

REFERENCES

1. Babcock, G. J., D. Hochberg, and A. D. Thorley-Lawson. 2000. The expression pattern of Epstein-Barr virus latent genes in vivo is dependent upon the differentiation stage of the infected B cell. Immunity 13:497–506.
2. Babcock, G. J., and D. A. Thorley-Lawson. 2000. Tonsillar memory B cells, latently infected with Epstein-Barr virus, express the restricted pattern of latent genes previously found only in Epstein-Barr virus-associated tumors. Proc. Natl. Acad. Sci. USA 97:12250–12255.
3. Bernasconi, M., C. Berger, J. A. Sigrist, A. Bonanomi, J. Sobek, F. K. Niggli, and D. Nadal. 2006. Quantitative profiling of housekeeping and Epstein-Barr virus gene transcription in Burkitt lymphoma cell lines using an oligonucleotide microarray. Virol. J. 3:43.
4. Bryant, H., and P. J. Farrell. 2002. Signal transduction and transcription factor modification during reactivation of Epstein-Barr virus from latency. J. Virol. 76:10290–10298.
5. Fruehling, S., S. K. Lee, R. Herrold, B. Frech, G. Laux, E. Kremmer, F. A. Grasser, and R. Longnecker. 1996. Identification of latent membrane protein 2A (LMP2A) domains essential for the LMP2A dominant-negative effect on B-lymphocyte surface immunoglobulin signal transduction. J. Virol. 70:6216–6226.
6. Fruehling, S., and R. Longnecker. 1997. The immunoreceptor tyrosine-based activation motif of Epstein-Barr virus LMP2A is essential for blocking BCR-mediated signal transduction. Virology 235:241–251.
7. Fukuda, M., and R. Longnecker. 2005. Epstein-Barr virus (EBV) latent membrane protein 2A regulates B-cell receptor-induced apoptosis and EBV reactivation through tyrosine phosphorylation. J. Virol. 79:8655–8660.
8. Gottschalk, S., C. M. Rooney, and H. E. Heslop. 2005. Post-transplant lymphoproliferative disorders. Annu. Rev. Med. 56:29–44.
9. Indra, A. K., X. Warot, J. Brocard, J. M. Bornert, J. H. Xiao, P. Chambon, and D. Metzger. 1999. Temporally-controlled site-specific mutagenesis in the basal layer of the epidermis: comparison of the recombinase activity of the tamoxifen-inducible Cre-ER(T) and Cre-ER(T2) recombinases. Nucleic Acids Res. 27:4324–4327.
10. Kim, P. S., and P. Arvan. 1998. Endocrinopathies in the family of endoplasmic reticulum (ER) storage diseases: disorders of protein trafficking and the role of ER molecular chaperones. Endocr. Rev. 19:173–202.
11. Kluiver, J., K. Kok, I. Pfeil, D. de Jong, T. Blokzijl, G. Harms, P. van der Vlies, A. Diepstra, C. Atayar, S. Poppema, R. Kuppers, and A. van den Berg. 2007. Global correlation of genome and transcriptome changes in classical Hodgkin lymphoma. Hematol. Oncol. 25:21–29.
12. Konishi, K., S. Maruo, H. Kato, and K. Takada. 2001. Role of Epstein-Barr virus-encoded latent membrane protein 2A on virus-induced immortalization and virus activation. J. Gen. Virol. 82:1451–1456.
13. Küppers, R., I. Schwering, A. Brauninger, K. Rajewsky, and M. L. Hansmann. 2002. Biology of Hodgkin's lymphoma. Ann. Oncol. 13(Suppl. 1):11–18.
14. Ladell, K., M. Dorner, L. Zauner, C. Berger, F. Zucol, M. Bernasconi, F. K. Niggli, R. F. Speck, and D. Nadal. 2007. Immune activation suppresses initiation of lytic Epstein-Barr virus infection. Cell. Microbiol. 9:2055–2069.
15. Longnecker, R., B. Druker, T. M. Roberts, and E. Kieff. 1991. An Epstein-Barr virus protein associated with cell growth transformation interacts with a tyrosine kinase. J. Virol. 65:3681–3692.
16. Longnecker, R., and E. Kieff. 1990. A second Epstein-Barr virus membrane protein (LMP2) is expressed in latent infection and colocalizes with LMP1. J. Virol. 64:2319–2326.
17. Lynch, D. T., J. S. Zimmerman, and D. T. Rowe. 2002. Epstein-Barr virus latent membrane protein 2B (LMP2B) co-localizes with LMP2A in perinuclear regions in transiently transfected cells. J. Gen. Virol. 83:1025–1035.
18. Matskova, L., I. Ernberg, T. Pawson, and G. Winberg. 2001. C-terminal domain of the Epstein-Barr virus LMP2A membrane protein contains a clustering signal. J. Virol. 75:10941–10949.
19. Meusser, B., C. Hirsch, E. Jarosch, and T. Sommer. 2005. ERAD: the long road to destruction. Nat. Cell Biol. 7:766–772.
20. Miller, C. L., A. L. Burkhardt, J. H. Lee, B. Stealey, R. Longnecker, J. B. Bolen, and E. Kieff. 1995. Integral membrane protein 2 of Epstein-Barr virus regulates reactivation from latency through dominant negative effects on protein-tyrosine kinases. Immunity 2:155–166.
21. Miller, C. L., J. H. Lee, E. Kieff, and R. Longnecker. 1994. An integral membrane protein (LMP2) blocks reactivation of Epstein-Barr virus from latency following surface immunoglobulin crosslinking. Proc. Natl. Acad. Sci. USA 91:772–776.
22. Miller, C. L., R. Longnecker, and E. Kieff. 1993. Epstein-Barr virus latent membrane protein 2A blocks calcium mobilization in B lymphocytes. J. Virol. 67:3087–3094.
23. Miller, G., and M. Lipman. 1973. Release of infectious Epstein-Barr virus by transformed marmoset leukocytes. Proc. Natl. Acad. Sci. USA 70:190–194.
24. Murray, P. G., and L. S. Young. 2002. The Role of the Epstein-Barr virus in human disease. Front. Biosci. 7:d519–d540.
25. Portis, T., and R. Longnecker. 2004. Epstein-Barr virus (EBV) LMP2A alters normal transcriptional regulation following B-cell receptor activation. Virology 318:524–533.
26. Portis, T., and R. Longnecker. 2004. Epstein-Barr virus (EBV) LMP2A mediates B-lymphocyte survival through constitutive activation of the Ras/PI3K/Akt pathway. Oncogene 23:8619–8628.
27. Rechsteiner, M. P., C. Berger, M. Weber, J. A. Sigrist, D. Nadal, and M. Bernasconi. 2007. Silencing of latent membrane protein 2B reduces susceptibility to activation of lytic Epstein-Barr virus in Burkitt's lymphoma Akata cells. J. Gen. Virol. 88:1454–1459.
28. Rickinson, A., and E. Kieff. 2001. Epstein-Barr virus, p. 2575–2627. In Knipe, D. M., P. M. Howley, D. E. Griffin, R. A. Lamb, M. A. Martin, B. Roizman, and S. E. Straus (ed.), Fields virology, 4th ed., vol. 2. Lippincott Williams & Wilkins, Philadelphia, PA.
29. Rovedo, M., and R. Longnecker. 2007. Epstein-Barr virus latent membrane protein 2B (LMP2B) modulates LMP2A activity. J. Virol. 81:84–94.
30. Rowe, D. T. 1999. Epstein-Barr virus immortalization and latency. Front. Biosci. 4:D346–D371.
31. Sample, J., D. Liebowitz, and E. Kieff. 1989. Two related Epstein-Barr virus membrane proteins are encoded by separate genes. J. Virol. 63:933–937.
32. Schaadt, E., B. Baier, J. Mautner, G. W. Bornkamm, and B. Adler. 2005. Epstein-Barr virus latent membrane protein 2A mimics B-cell receptor-dependent virus reactivation. J. Gen. Virol. 86:551–559.
33. Schaefer, B. C., T. C. Mitchell, J. W. Kappler, and P. Marrack. 2001. A novel family of retroviral vectors for the rapid production of complex stable cell lines. Anal. Biochem. 297:86–93.
34. Sugden, B., and W. Mark. 1977. Clonal transformation of adult human leukocytes by Epstein-Barr virus. J. Virol. 23:503–508.
35. Swart, R., I. K. Ruf, J. Sample, and R. Longnecker. 2000. Latent membrane protein 2A-mediated effects on the phosphatidylinositol 3-kinase/Akt pathway. J. Virol. 74:10838–10845.
36. Takada, K. 1984. Cross-linking of cell surface immunoglobulins induces Epstein-Barr virus in Burkitt lymphoma lines. Int. J. Cancer 33:27–32.
37. Tomaszewski-Flick, M. J., and D. T. Rowe. 2007. Minimal protein domain requirements for the intracellular localization and self-aggregation of Epstein-Barr virus latent membrane protein 2. Virus Genes 35:225–234.
38. Young, L. S., and P. G. Murray. 2003. Epstein-Barr virus and oncogenesis: from latent genes to tumours. Oncogene 22:5108–5121.
39. Yuan, J., E. Cahir-McFarland, B. Zhao, and E. Kieff. 2006. Virus and cell RNAs expressed during Epstein-Barr virus replication. J. Virol. 80:2548–2565.

7. Discussion

7.1 Induction of lytic EBV infection as treatment in clinics

Although there is good response to chemotherapy from BL and HL and as well encouraging prognosis after treatment, the side effects of using chemical agents are often dramatic. Thus, other approaches to eliminate these tumors were taken into account.

The fact, that most of these tumors contain EBV in the vast majority of the tumor cells (Table 3), gave rise to the formulation of new possible tumor therapies. Prevention and treatment of EBV-associated tumors have focussed on counteracting the transforming effects of established latent EBV infection, i.e., the proliferation and expansion of EBV transformed cells *in vivo* using cytotoxic drugs, anti-B-cell antibodies, reduction of iatrogenic immunosuppression, or EBV-specific cytotoxic T lymphocytes. Unfortunately, these approaches are as well burdened with significant untoward effects including ample destruction of non-malignant cells, allograft rejection, life-threatening secondary infections, and technical as well as logistic hurdles. Furthermore, the efficiency is far from being satisfactory.

Another approach, i.e., the one to induce lytic EBV infection was investigated in this thesis. The DNA methyl transferase inhibitor (DNMTI) Zebularine has previously been shown to specifically induce cell death in tumor cells by demethylation of silenced tumor suppressor genes. We focused on the demethylation of silenced hypermethylated EBV genes to activate lytic infection by Zebularine which would have been an elegant way to kill all EBV-harboring tumor cells. Unfortunately, we could not show induction of lytic EBV infection in the BL cell line Akata using Zebularine, in contrast to control treatments with 5-Azacytidine resulting in cell death due to lytic EBV activation. Additionally, we positively verified demethylation activity of Zebularine by reactivation of *E*-cadherin expression which is normally silenced in Akata cells. Summarizing these findings, the promising new DNMTI Zebularine seems not to be an appropriate drug for the treatment of EBV-positive tumors. For more detailed information and discussion see section 6.1.

7.2 Induction of lytic EBV infection by LMP2B as treatment in clinics

Induction of lytic EBV infection via gene manipulation seems to be more promising than chemical induction as discussed in paragraph 8.1. In our studies, we could demonstrate higher lytic EBV infection in BL Akata cells after BCR cross-linking when LMP2B was overexpressed *in vitro* (see sections 6.3). These results reveal a possible target for clinical therapy of EBV-associated tumors. However, there are many questions to be resolved first. Primarily, the effect of LMP2B has to be validated in a mouse model. Such a mouse model is, e.g., a SCID (Severe Combined Immuno Deficiency) mouse model in which human BL Akata cells overexpressing LMP2B are injected and grow due to the lack of an intact immune response. After xenotransplantation, the growing tumor will be stimulated with anti-IgG as described in the *in vitro* experiments (section 6). If overexpression of LMP2B has the same effect *in vivo* as observed *in vitro*, the tumor growth should decrease and vanish due to lytic EBV infection and tumor cell death.

After this proof of principle in a mouse model, the next step would be to find an appropriate delivery system for LMP2B to the tumor *in vivo*. There are various options for the introduction of a foreign gene into a host and its integration into the genome. Among them (i) injection of naked or coated LMP2B with a gene-gun directly into the tumor tissue, (ii) infection of host cells with an attenuated virus expressing LMP2B, or (iii) completely artificial generated transport vehicles consisting of an outer membrane with surface receptors specific for B-cell homing and a 'genome' containing LMP2B and viral components for integration. The method of choice will depend on the progress in overcoming the technical hurdles which are still manifold in gene therapy.

8. Conclusions and outlook

Taken together, the results presented in this PhD thesis shed new light on the regulation of latent and lytic EBV infection. Most importantly, new functions as a rheostat of LMP2A could be assigned to LMP2B and could be integrated into a model describing the development of EBV infected B-cells and B-cell derived lymphomas. The importance of a careful regulation of the expression levels of LMP2A and LMP2B depending on the physiological situation seems to be evident and shifting to either one or the other side of the balance determines the fate of the infected B-cell harboring EBV. So far, the factors which act as sensors for differential expression levels of LMP2B are not determined. It will be an interesting and challenging task to elucidate the regulatory mechanisms of the expression of LMP2B.

Finally, once the function of LMP2B is defined *in vitro* and *in vivo*, the step towards tailoring new therapeutic approaches in the treatment of EBV associated lymphomas using LMP2B as an inducer of lytic EBV infection comes into reach.

9. Literature

1. Zimet, G.D., et al. (2008) Appropriate Use of Cervical Cancer Vaccine. Annu Rev Med 59, 223-236
2. Hilleman, M.R. (1998) Overview of viruses, cancer, and vaccines in concept and in reality. Recent Results Cancer Res 154, 345-362
3. Kao, J.H., and Chen, D.S. (2002) Global control of hepatitis B virus infection. Lancet Infect Dis 2, 395-403
4. Hanahan, D., and Weinberg, R.A. (2000) The hallmarks of cancer. Cell 100, 57-70
5. Dent, R., and Warner, E. (2007) Screening for hereditary breast cancer. Semin Oncol 34, 392-400
6. Knudson, A.G., Jr. (1971) Mutation and cancer: statistical study of retinoblastoma. Proc Natl Acad Sci U S A 68, 820-823
7. Boccardo, E., and Villa, L.L. (2007) Viral origins of human cancer. Curr Med Chem 14, 2526-2539
8. Matsuoka, M., and Jeang, K.T. (2007) Human T-cell leukaemia virus type 1 (HTLV-1) infectivity and cellular transformation. Nat Rev Cancer 7, 270-280
9. Soni, V., et al. (2007) LMP1 TRAFficking activates growth and survival pathways. Adv Exp Med Biol 597, 173-187
10. Rickinson, A., and Kieff, E. (2001) Epstein-Barr Virus. In Fields Virology (4th edn) (Knipe, D.M., and Howley, P.M., eds), 2575-2627, Lippincott Williams & Wilkins Publishers
11. Klein, G. (1994) Epstein-Barr virus strategy in normal and neoplastic B cells. Cell 77, 791-793
12. Thompson, M.P., and Kurzrock, R. (2004) Epstein-Barr virus and cancer. Clin Cancer Res 10, 803-821
13. Hochberg, D., et al. (2004) Demonstration of the Burkitt's lymphoma Epstein-Barr virus phenotype in dividing latently infected memory cells in vivo. Proc Natl Acad Sci U S A 101, 239-244
14. Thorley-Lawson, D.A., and Gross, A. (2004) Persistence of the Epstein-Barr virus and the origins of associated lymphomas. N Engl J Med 350, 1328-1337
15. Epstein, M.A., et al. (1964) Virus Particles In Cultured Lymphoblasts From Burkitt's Lymphoma. Lancet 15, 702-703

16. Rochford, R., *et al.* (2005) Endemic Burkitt's lymphoma: a polymicrobial disease? *Nat Rev Microbiol* 3, 182-187
17. Allday, M.J., and Crawford, D.H. (1988) Role of epithelium in EBV persistence and pathogenesis of B-cell tumours. *Lancet* 1, 855-857
18. Miyashita, E.M., *et al.* (1997) Identification of the site of Epstein-Barr virus persistence in vivo as a resting B cell.[erratum appears in J Virol 1998 Nov;72(11):9419]. *J. Virol.* 71, 4882-4891
19. Babcock, G.J., *et al.* (1998) EBV persistence in memory B cells in vivo. *Immunity* 9, 395-404
20. Clemens, M.J. (2006) Epstein-Barr virus: inhibition of apoptosis as a mechanism of cell transformation. *Int J Biochem Cell Biol* 38, 164-169
21. Clemens, M.J., and Elia, A. (1997) The double-stranded RNA-dependent protein kinase PKR: structure and function. *J Interferon Cytokine Res* 17, 503-524
22. Clemens, M.J. (2004) Targets and mechanisms for the regulation of translation in malignant transformation. *Oncogene* 23, 3180-3188
23. Fruehling, S., and Longnecker, R. (1997) The immunoreceptor tyrosine-based activation motif of Epstein-Barr virus LMP2A is essential for blocking BCR-mediated signal transduction. *Virology* 235, 241-251
24. Rowe, D.T. (1999) Epstein-Barr virus immortalization and latency. *Front Biosci* 4, D346-371
25. Cesarman, E. (2002) Epstein-Barr virus (EBV) and lymphomagenesis. *Front. Biosci.* 7, e58-65
26. Brady, G., *et al.* (2007) Epstein-Barr virus and Burkitt lymphoma. *J Clin Pathol* 60, 1397-1402
27. Cherney, B.W., *et al.* (1997) Role of the p53 tumor suppressor gene in the tumorigenicity of Burkitt's lymphoma cells. *Cancer Res* 57, 2508-2515
28. Clybouw, C., *et al.* (2005) EBV infection of human B lymphocytes leads to down-regulation of Bim expression: relationship to resistance to apoptosis. *J Immunol* 175, 2968-2973
29. Farrell, P.J., *et al.* (1991) p53 is frequently mutated in Burkitt's lymphoma cell lines. *Embo J* 10, 2879-2887
30. Kamranvar, S.A., *et al.* (2007) Epstein-Barr virus promotes genomic instability in Burkitt's lymphoma. *Oncogene* 26, 5115-5123

31. Kuhn-Hallek, I., *et al.* (1995) Expression of recombination activating genes (RAG-1 and RAG-2) in Epstein-Barr virus-bearing B cells. *Blood* 85, 1289-1299
32. Jox, A., *et al.* (1997) Integration of Epstein-Barr virus in Burkitt's lymphoma cells leads to a region of enhanced chromosome instability. *Ann Oncol* 8 Suppl 2, 131-135
33. Gualandi, G., *et al.* (2001) Enhancement of genetic instability in human B cells by Epstein-Barr virus latent infection. *Mutagenesis* 16, 203-208
34. Kelly, K., and Knox, K.A. (1995) Differential regulatory effects of cAMP-elevating agents on human normal and neoplastic B cell functional response following ligation of surface immunoglobulin and CD40. *Cell Immunol* 166, 93-102
35. Takada, K. (1984) Cross-linking of cell surface immunoglobulins induces Epstein-Barr virus in Burkitt lymphoma lines. *Int J Cancer* 33, 27-32
36. Chene, A., *et al.* (2007) A molecular link between malaria and Epstein-Barr virus reactivation. *PLoS pathogens* 3, e80
37. Brauninger, A., *et al.* (2006) Molecular biology of Hodgkin's and Reed/Sternberg cells in Hodgkin's lymphoma. *Int J Cancer* 118, 1853-1861
38. Kuppers, R., *et al.* (2002) Biology of Hodgkin's lymphoma. *Ann Oncol* 13 Suppl 1, 11-18
39. Cuomo, L., *et al.* (1993) Selective induction of allostimulatory capacity after 5-azaC treatment of EBV carrying but not EBV negative Burkitt lymphoma cell lines. *Mol Immunol* 30, 441-450
40. Daibata, M., *et al.* (2005) Induction of lytic Epstein-Barr virus (EBV) infection by synergistic action of rituximab and dexamethasone renders EBV-positive lymphoma cells more susceptible to ganciclovir cytotoxicity in vitro and in vivo. *J Virol* 79, 5875-5879
41. Esteller, M. (2005) DNA methylation and cancer therapy: new developments and expectations. *Curr Opin Oncol* 17, 55-60
42. Lemaire, M., *et al.* (2005) Enhancement of antineoplastic action of 5-aza-2'-deoxycytidine by zebularine on L1210 leukemia. *Anticancer Drugs* 16, 301-308
43. Inman, G.J., *et al.* (2001) Activators of the Epstein-Barr virus lytic program concomitantly induce apoptosis, but lytic gene expression protects from cell death. *J Virol* 75, 2400-2410
44. Hsu, C.H., *et al.* (2002) Induction of Epstein-Barr virus (EBV) reactivation in Raji cells by doxorubicin and cisplatin. *Anticancer Res* 22, 4065-4071

45. Feng, W.H., *et al.* (2004) Lytic induction therapy for Epstein-Barr virus-positive B-cell lymphomas. *J Virol* 78, 1893-1902
46. Feng, W.H., *et al.* (2004) Reactivation of latent Epstein-Barr virus by methotrexate: a potential contributor to methotrexate-associated lymphomas. *J Natl Cancer Inst* 96, 1691-1702
47. Rao, S.P., *et al.* (2007) Zebularine reactivates silenced E-cadherin but unlike 5-Azacytidine does not induce switching from latent to lytic Epstein-Barr virus infection in Burkitt's lymphoma Akata cells. *Mol Cancer* 6, 3
48. Miller, G., *et al.* (2007) Lytic cycle switches of oncogenic human gammaherpesviruses(1). *Adv Cancer Res* 97, 81-109
49. Jung, E.J., *et al.* (2007) Lytic induction and apoptosis of Epstein-Barr virus-associated gastric cancer cell line with epigenetic modifiers and ganciclovir. *Cancer Lett* 247, 77-83
50. Cheng, J.C., *et al.* (2003) Inhibition of DNA methylation and reactivation of silenced genes by zebularine. *J Natl Cancer Inst* 95, 399-409
51. Zhou, L., *et al.* (2002) Zebularine: a novel DNA methylation inhibitor that forms a covalent complex with DNA methyltransferases. *J Mol Biol* 321, 591-599
52. Cihak, A. (1974) Biological effects of 5-azacytidine in eukaryotes. *Oncology* 30, 405-422
53. Cheng, J.C., *et al.* (2004) Preferential response of cancer cells to zebularine. *Cancer Cell* 6, 151-158
54. Sun, C.C., and Thorley-Lawson, D.A. (2007) Plasma cell-specific transcription factor XBP-1s binds to and transactivates the Epstein-Barr virus BZLF1 promoter. *J Virol* 81, 13566-13577
55. Bhende, P.M., *et al.* (2007) X-box-binding protein 1 activates lytic Epstein-Barr virus gene expression in combination with protein kinase D. *J Virol* 81, 7363-7370
56. Thorley-Lawson, D.A. (2001) Epstein-Barr virus: exploiting the immune system. *Nat Rev Immunol* 1, 75-82
57. Longnecker, R. (2000) Epstein-Barr virus latency: LMP2, a regulator or means for Epstein-Barr virus persistence? *Adv Cancer Res* 79, 175-200
58. Rechsteiner, M.P., *et al.* (2007) Silencing of latent membrane protein 2B reduces susceptibility to activation of lytic Epstein-Barr virus in Burkitt's lymphoma Akata cells. *J Gen Virol* 88, 1454-1459

59. Rechsteiner, M.P., *et al.* (2007) Latent Membrane Protein 2B Regulates Susceptibility to Induction of Lytic Epstein-Barr Virus Infection. *J Virol*
60. Rovedo, M., and Longnecker, R. (2007) Epstein-barr virus latent membrane protein 2B (LMP2B) modulates LMP2A activity. *J Virol* 81, 84-94

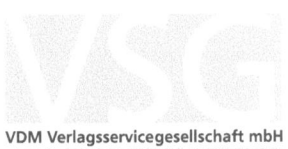

VDM Verlagsservicegesellschaft mbH

Die VDM Verlagsservicegesellschaft sucht für wissenschaftliche Verlage abgeschlossene und herausragende

Dissertationen, Habilitationen, Diplomarbeiten, Master Theses, Magisterarbeiten usw.

für die kostenlose Publikation als Fachbuch.

Sie verfügen über eine Arbeit, die hohen inhaltlichen und formalen Ansprüchen genügt, und haben Interesse an einer honorarvergüteten Publikation?

Dann senden Sie bitte erste Informationen über sich und Ihre Arbeit per Email an *info@vdm-vsg.de*.

Sie erhalten kurzfristig unser Feedback!

VDM Verlagsservicegesellschaft mbH
Dudweiler Landstr. 99   Telefon +49 681 3720 174
D - 66123 Saarbrücken   Fax   +49 681 3720 1749
www.vdm-vsg.de

Die VDM Verlagsservicegesellschaft mbH vertritt

  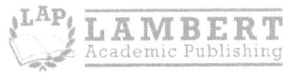 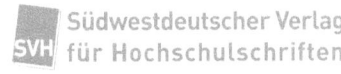

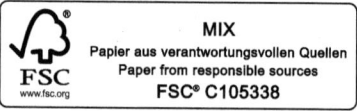

Printed by Books on Demand GmbH, Norderstedt / Germany